Best Mom Ever Coloring Book

© 2018 Rhonda Taylor

All Rights Reserved.

This book or parts thereof may not be reproduced in any form, stored in any retrieval system, or transmitted in any form by any means—electronic, mechanical, photocopy, recording, or otherwise—without prior written permission of the Publisher

Color Test Page

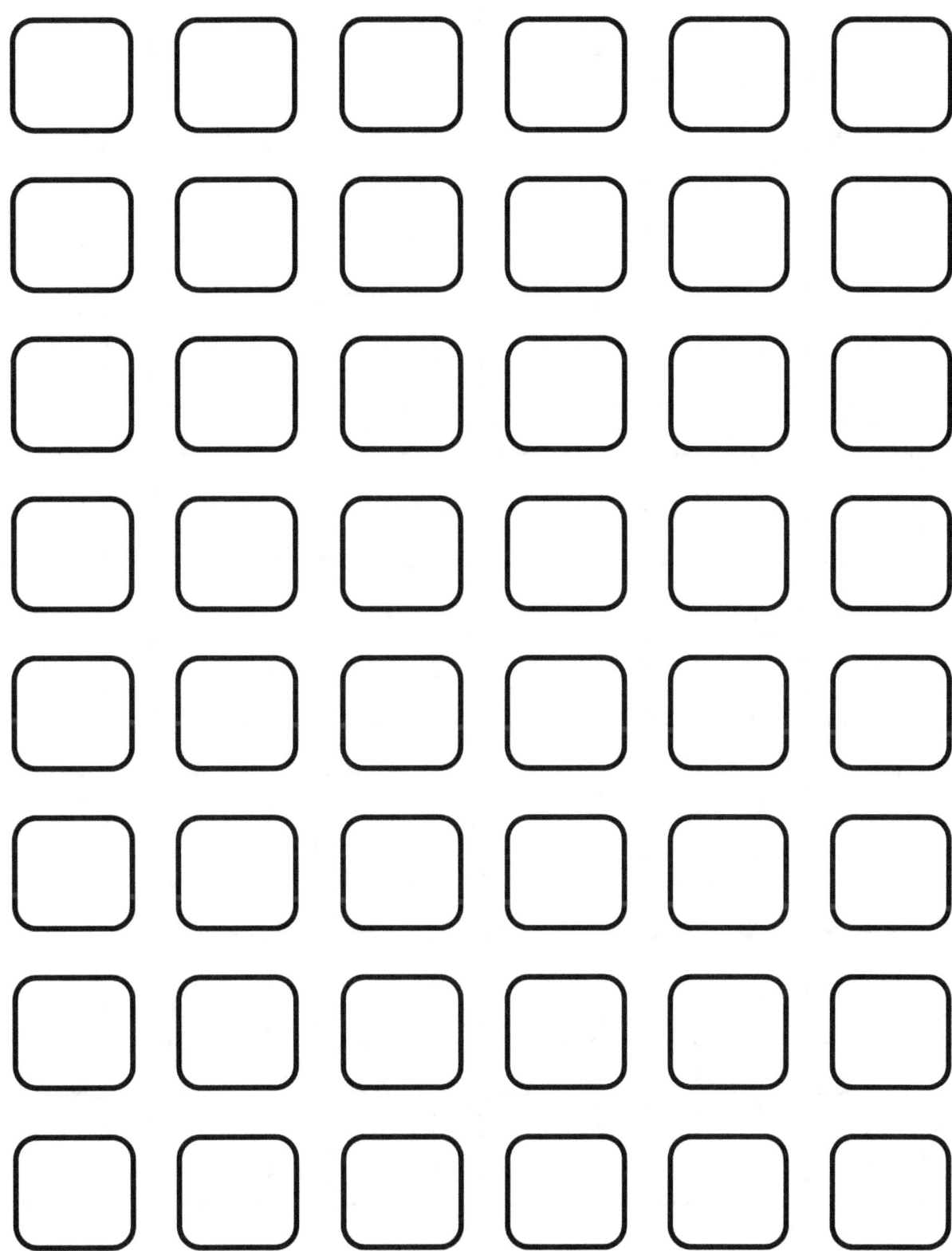

Color Test Page

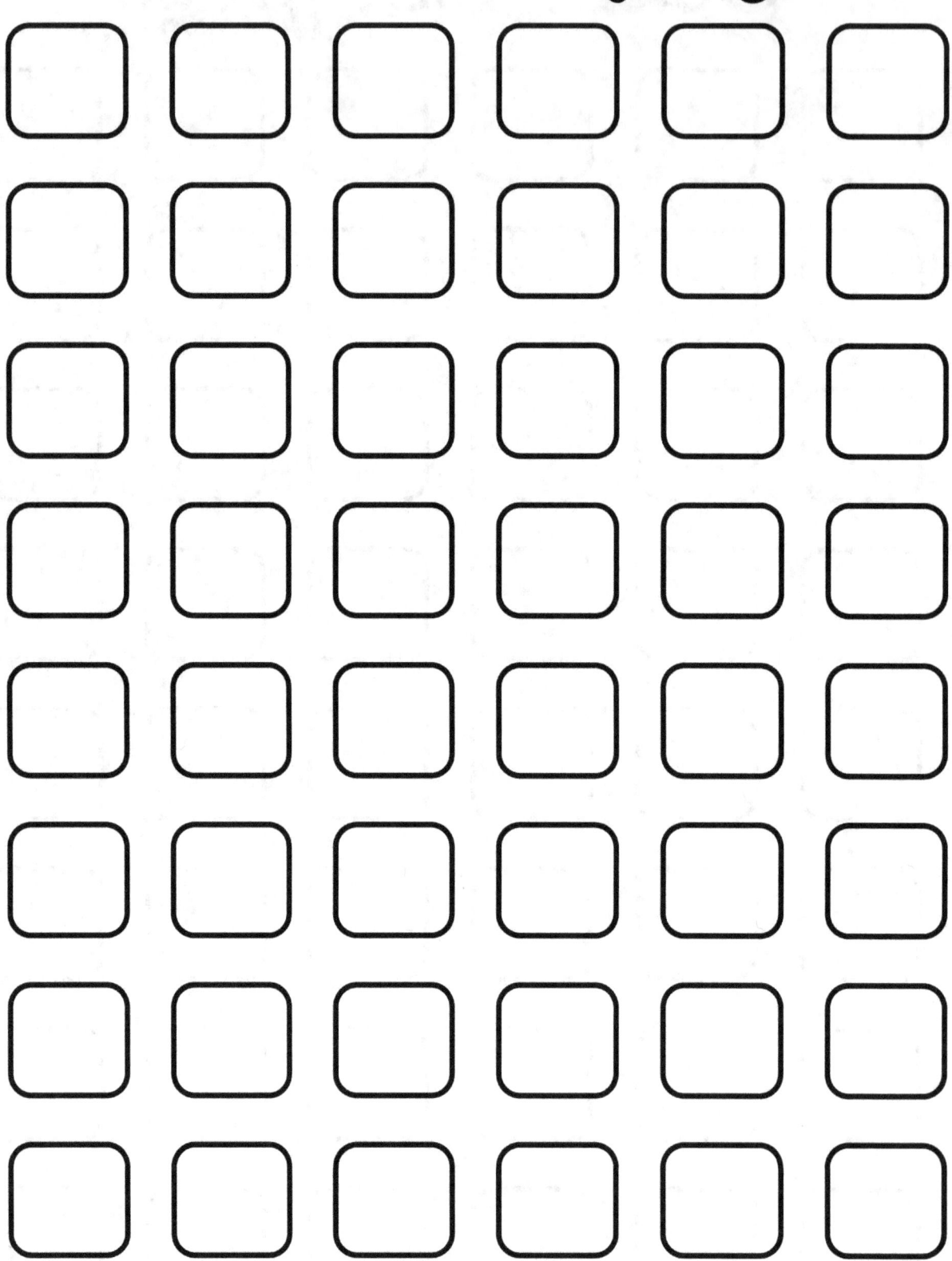

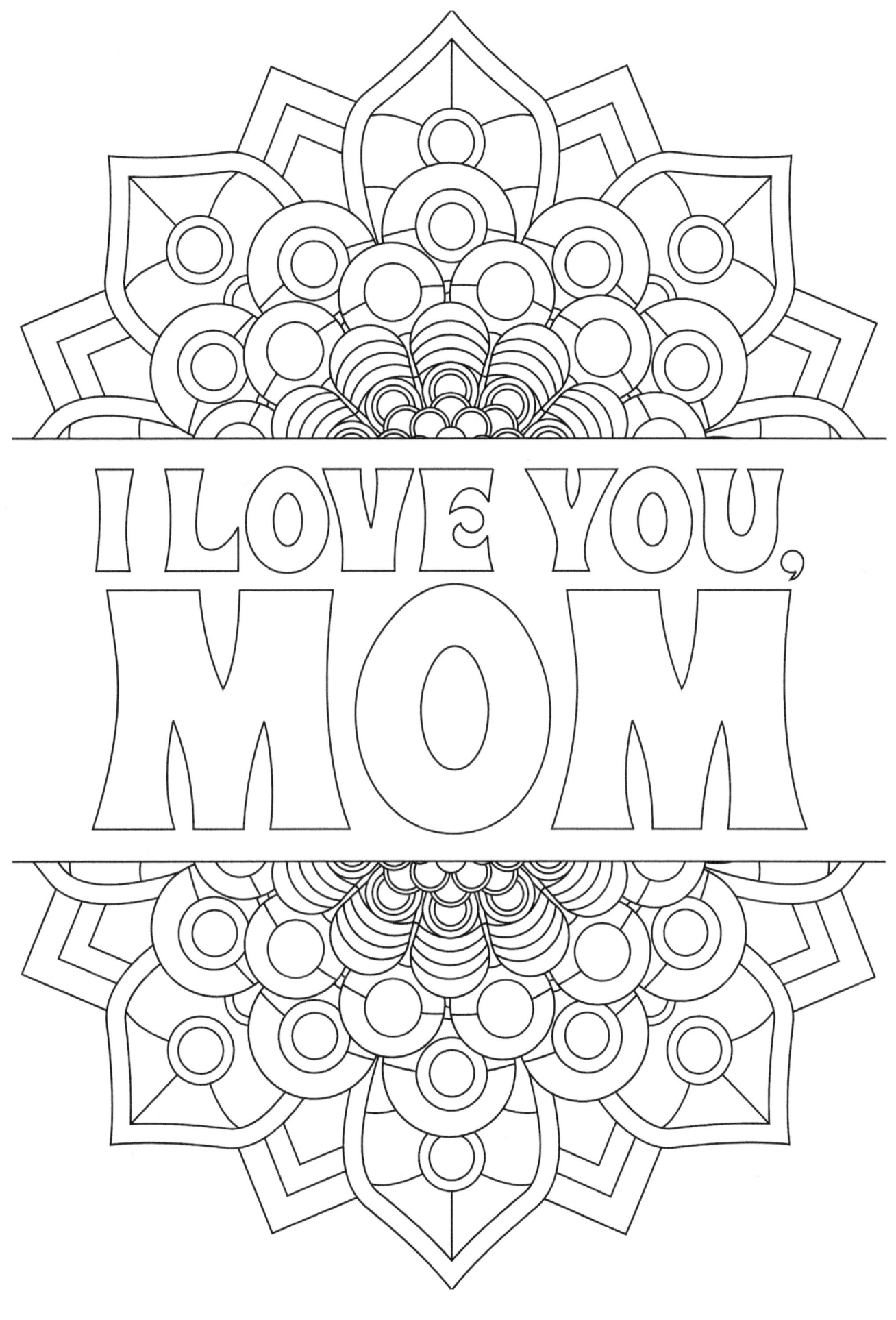

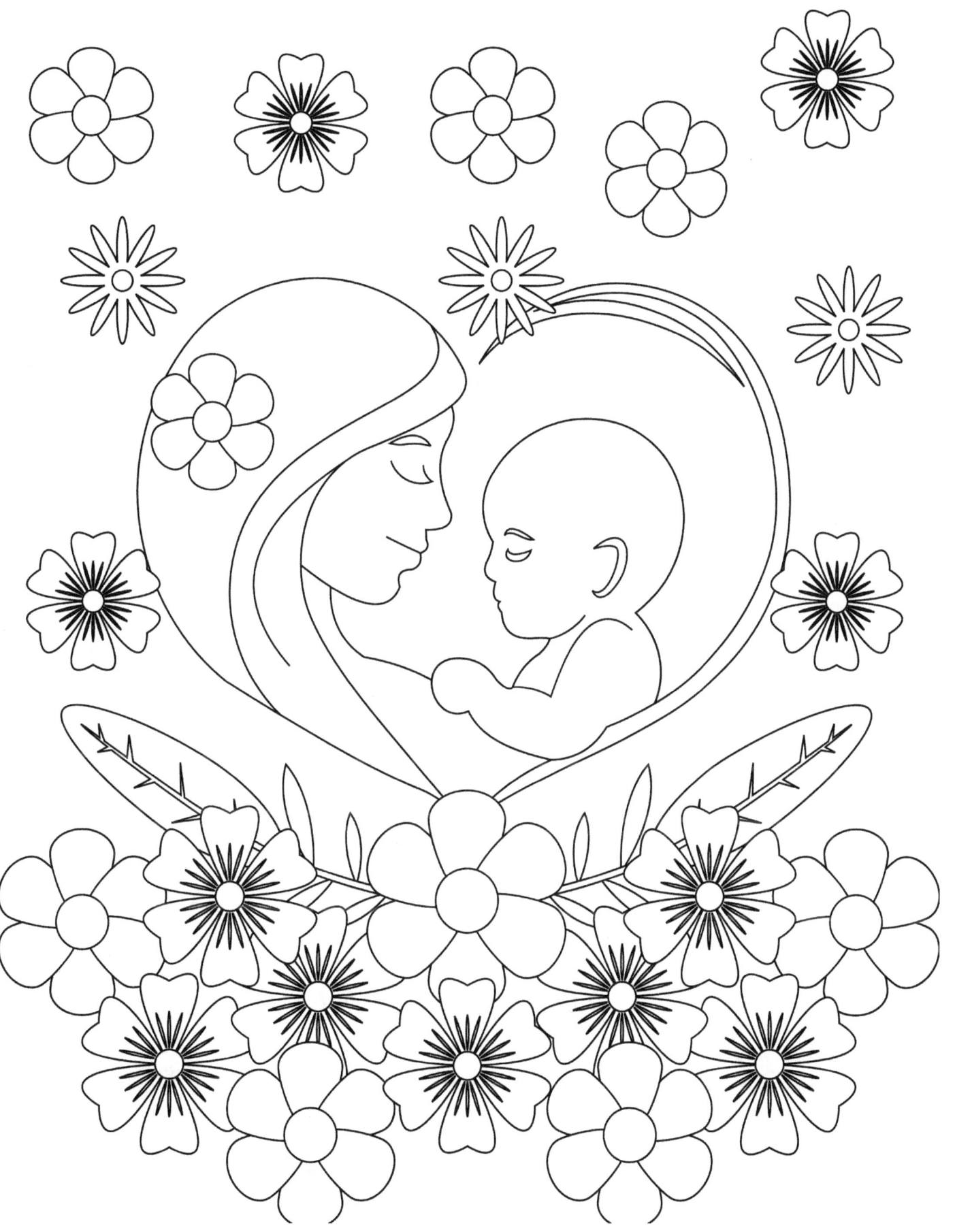

Life doesn't come with a manual,

IT COMES WITH A MOTHER

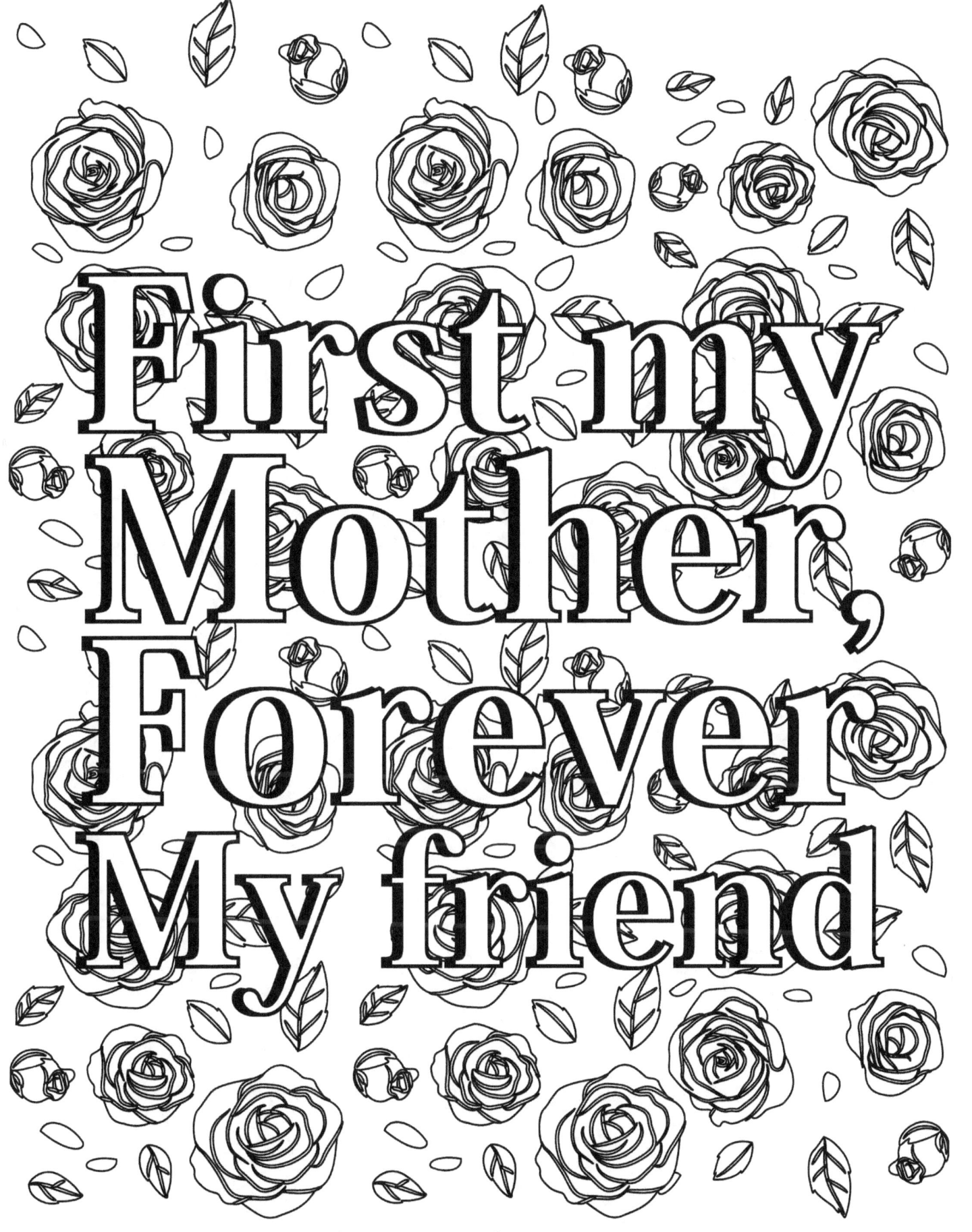

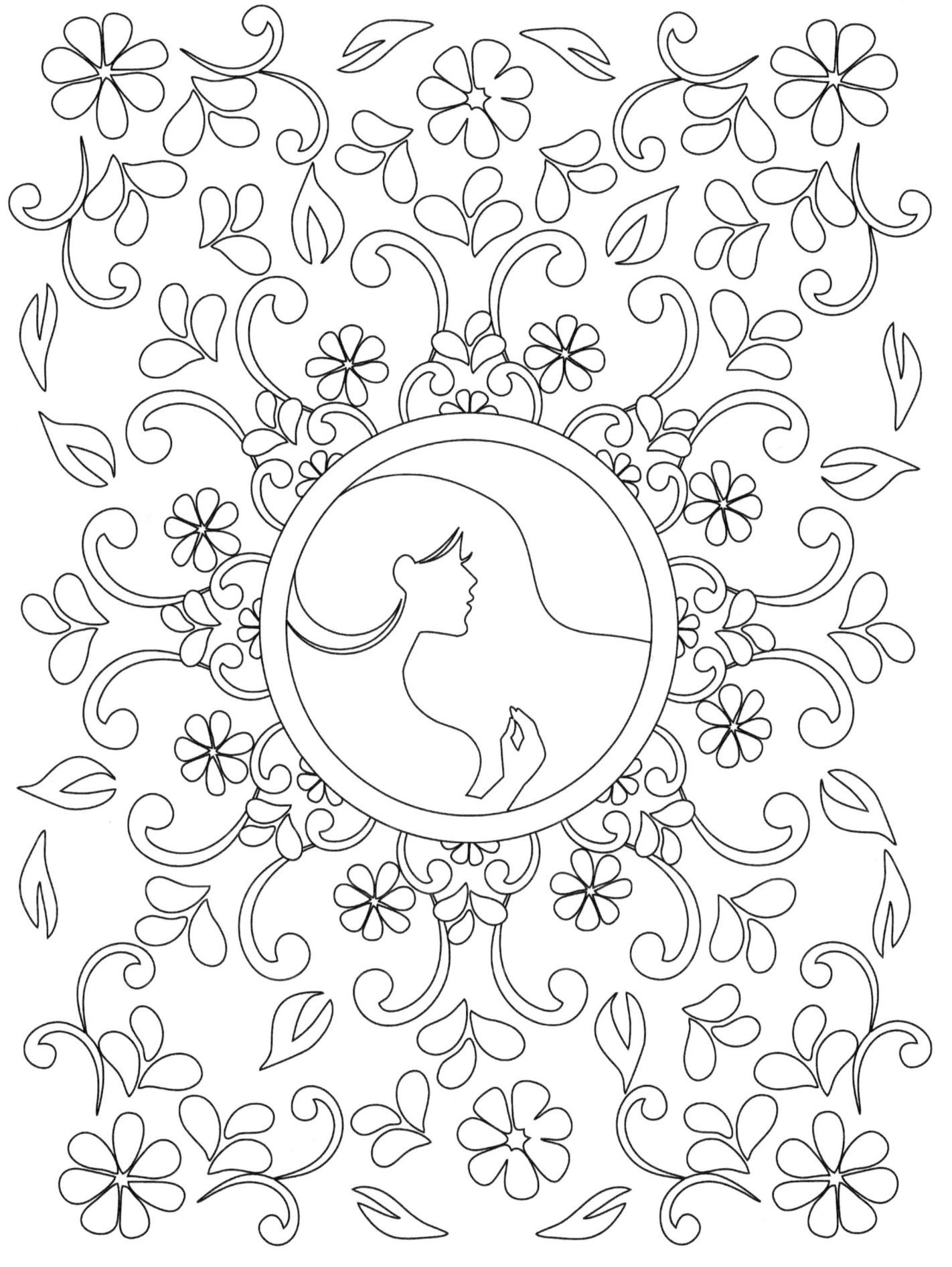

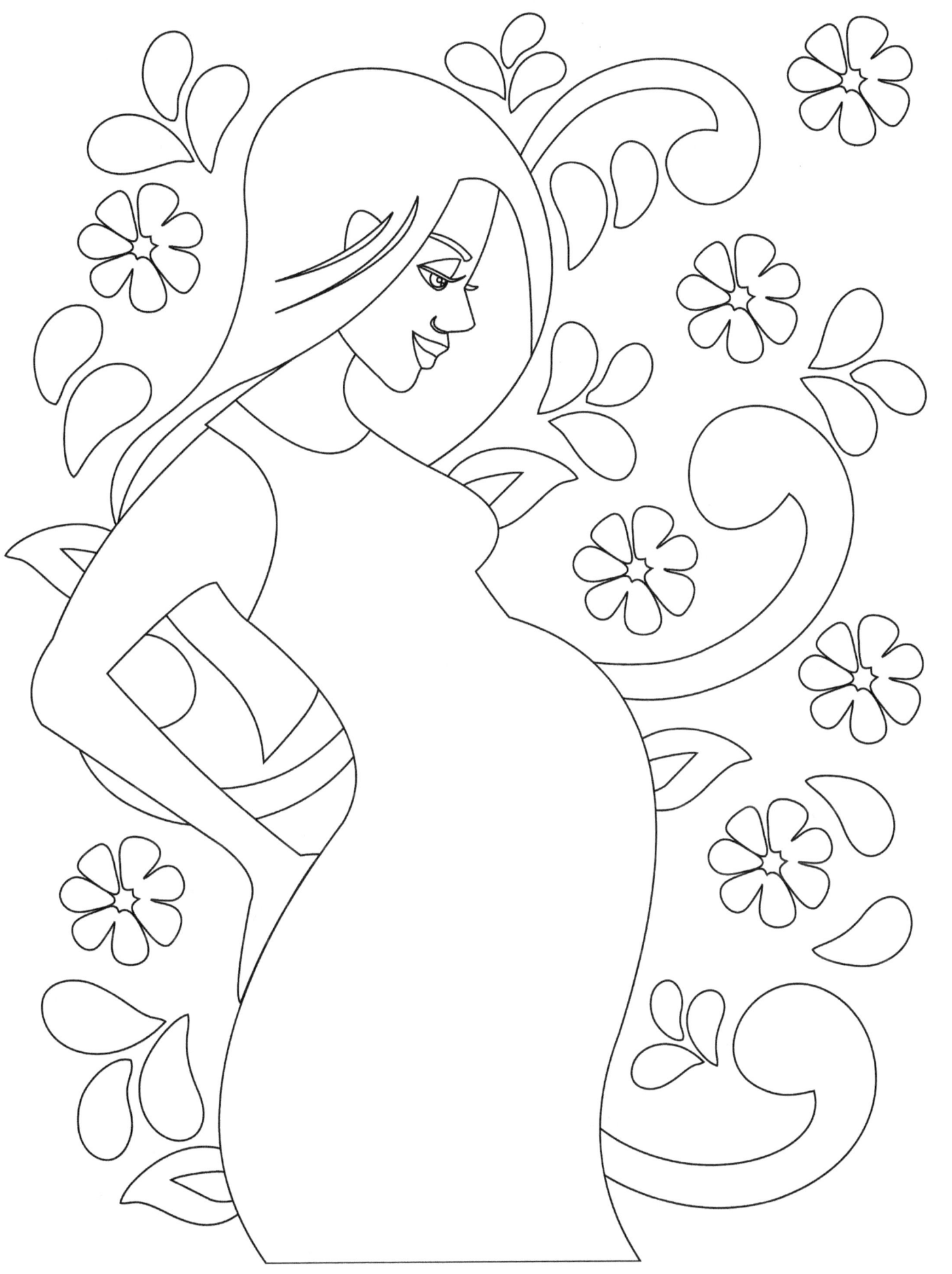

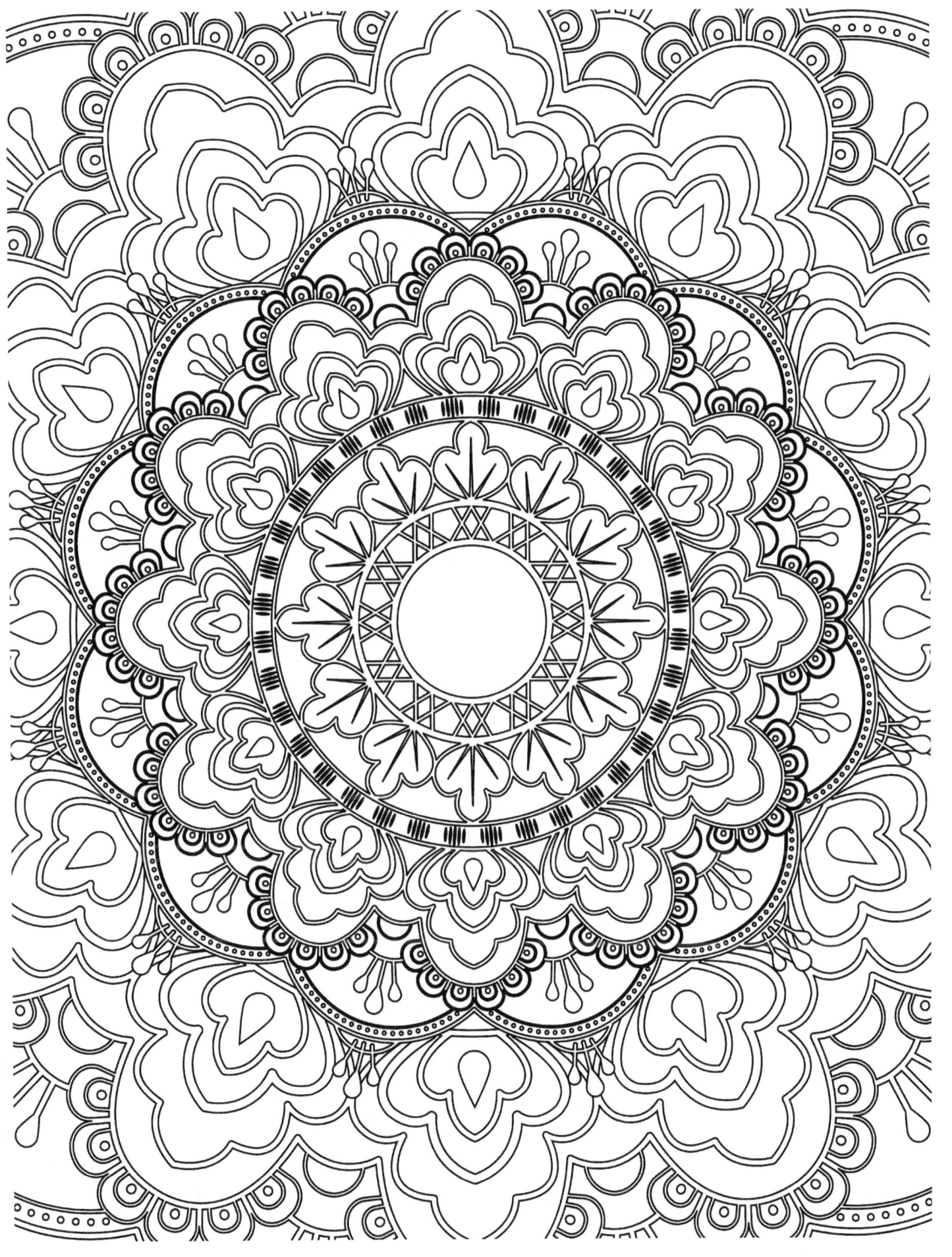

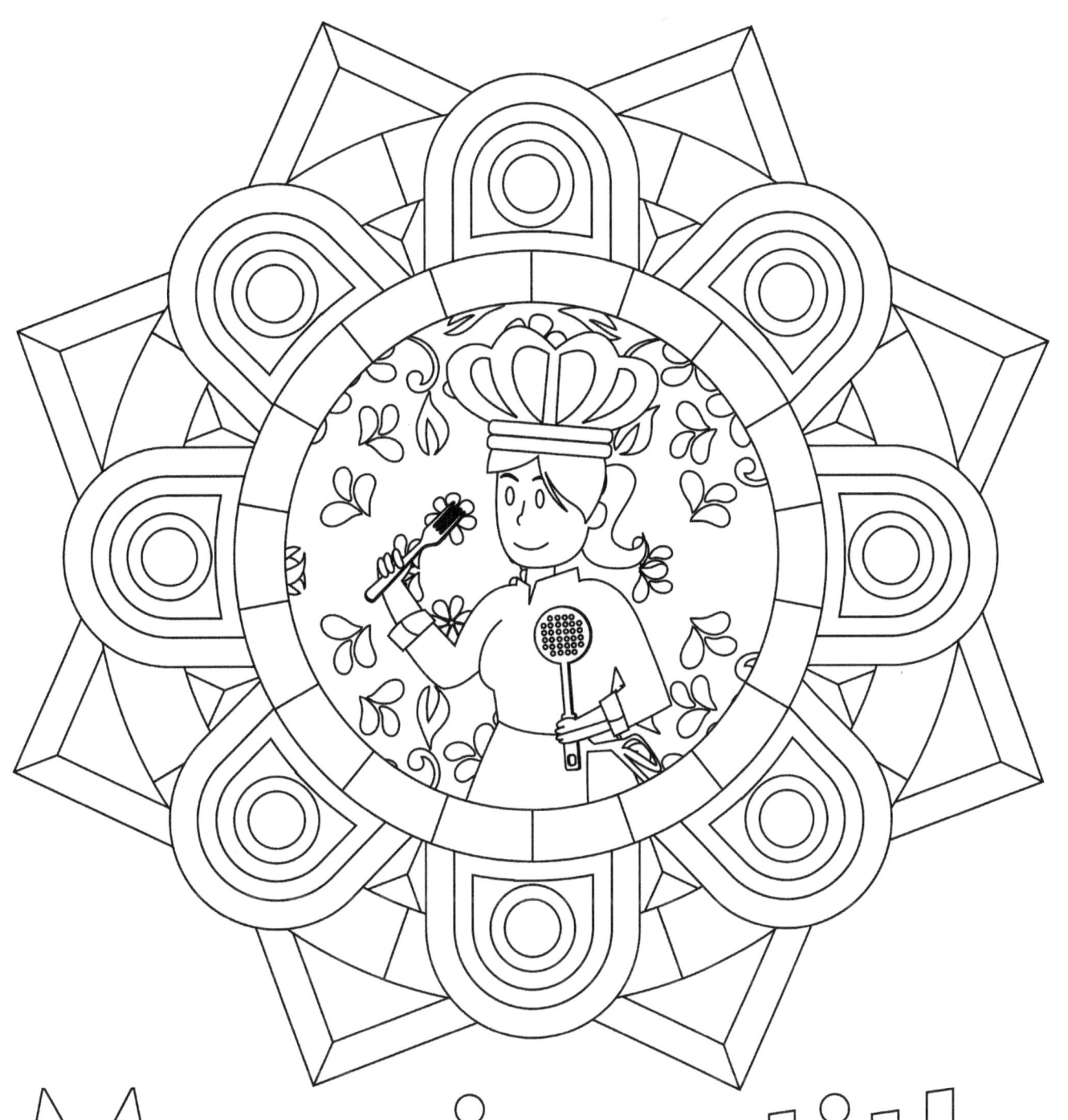

Mom is a title just above Queen

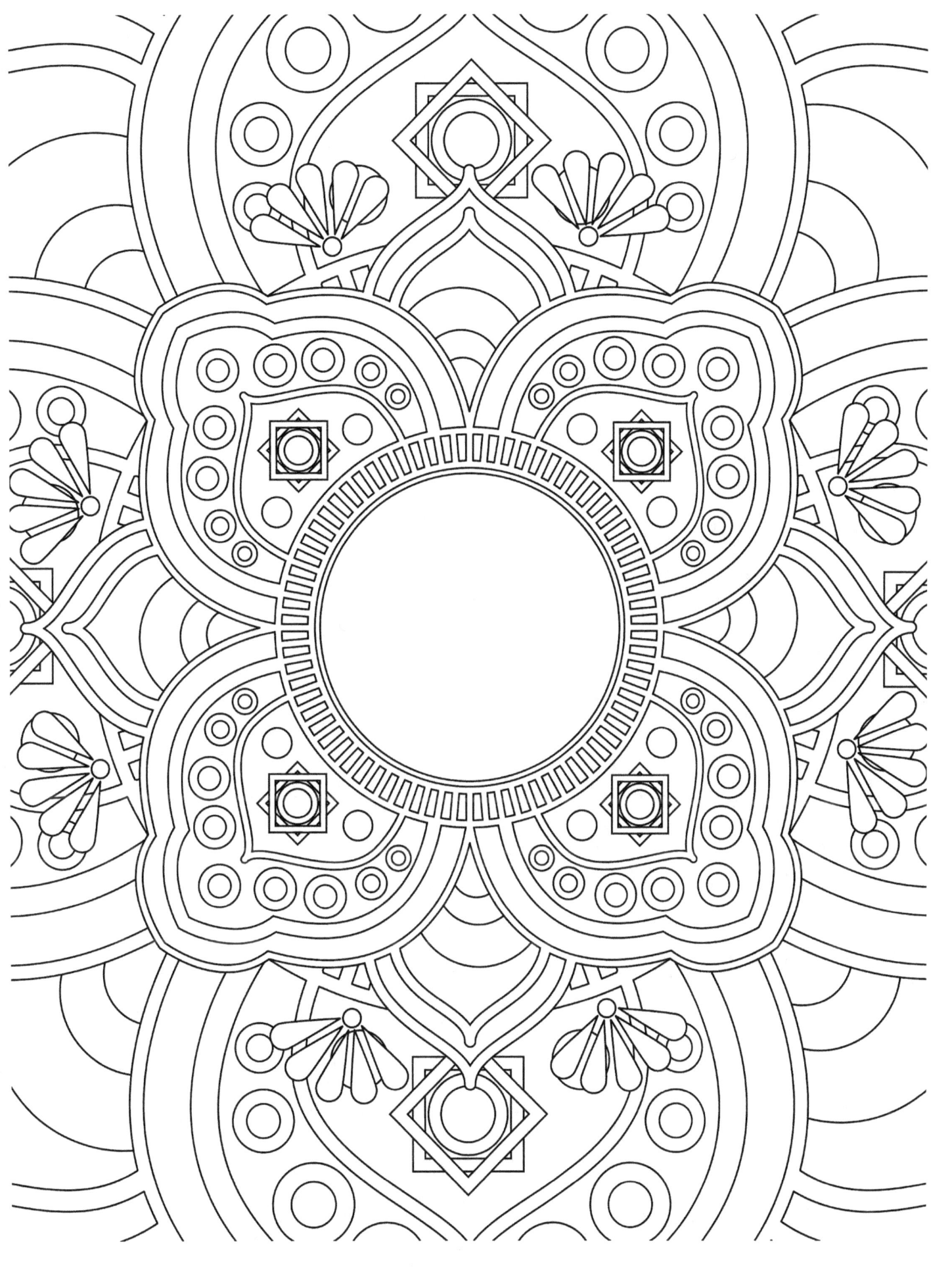

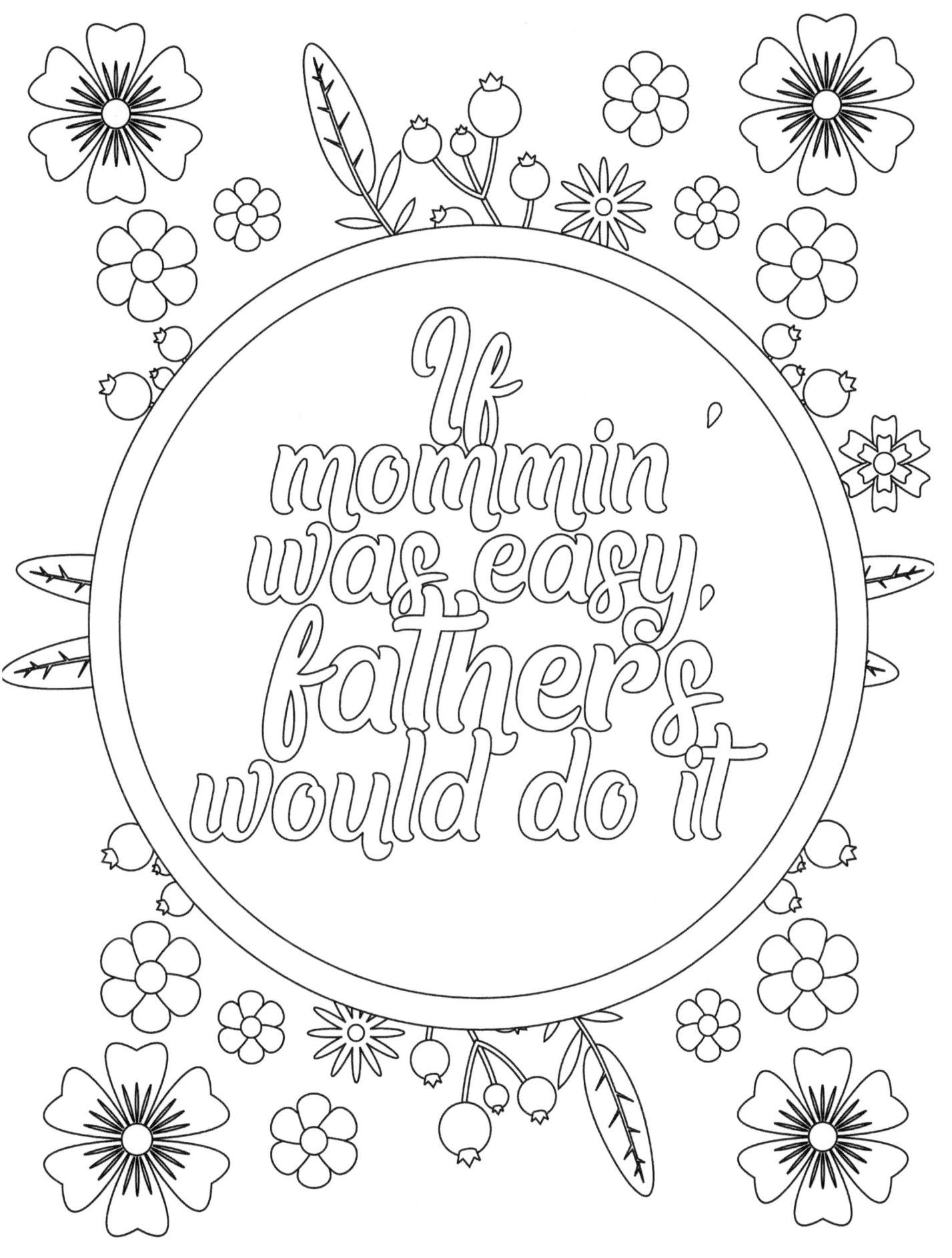

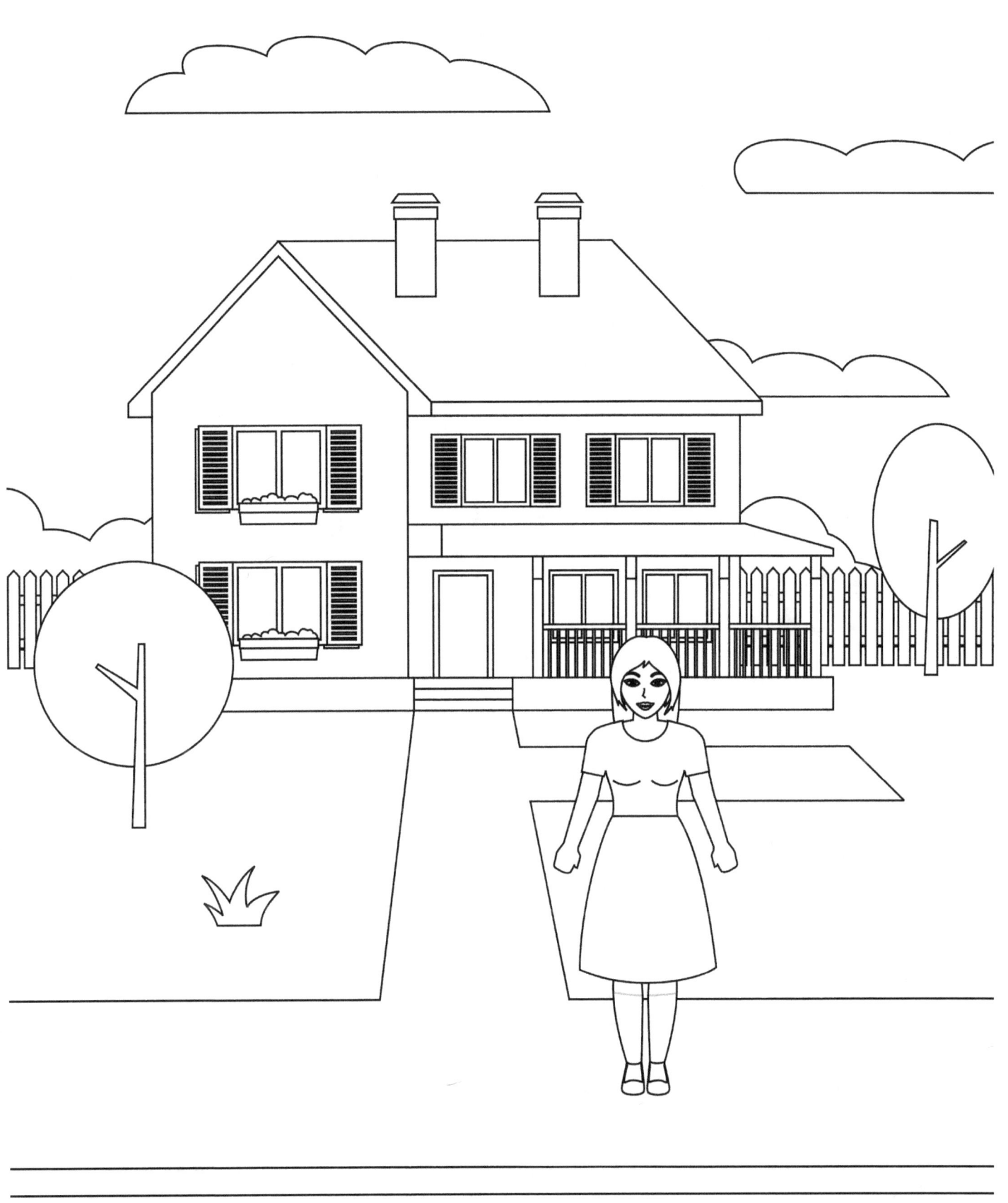

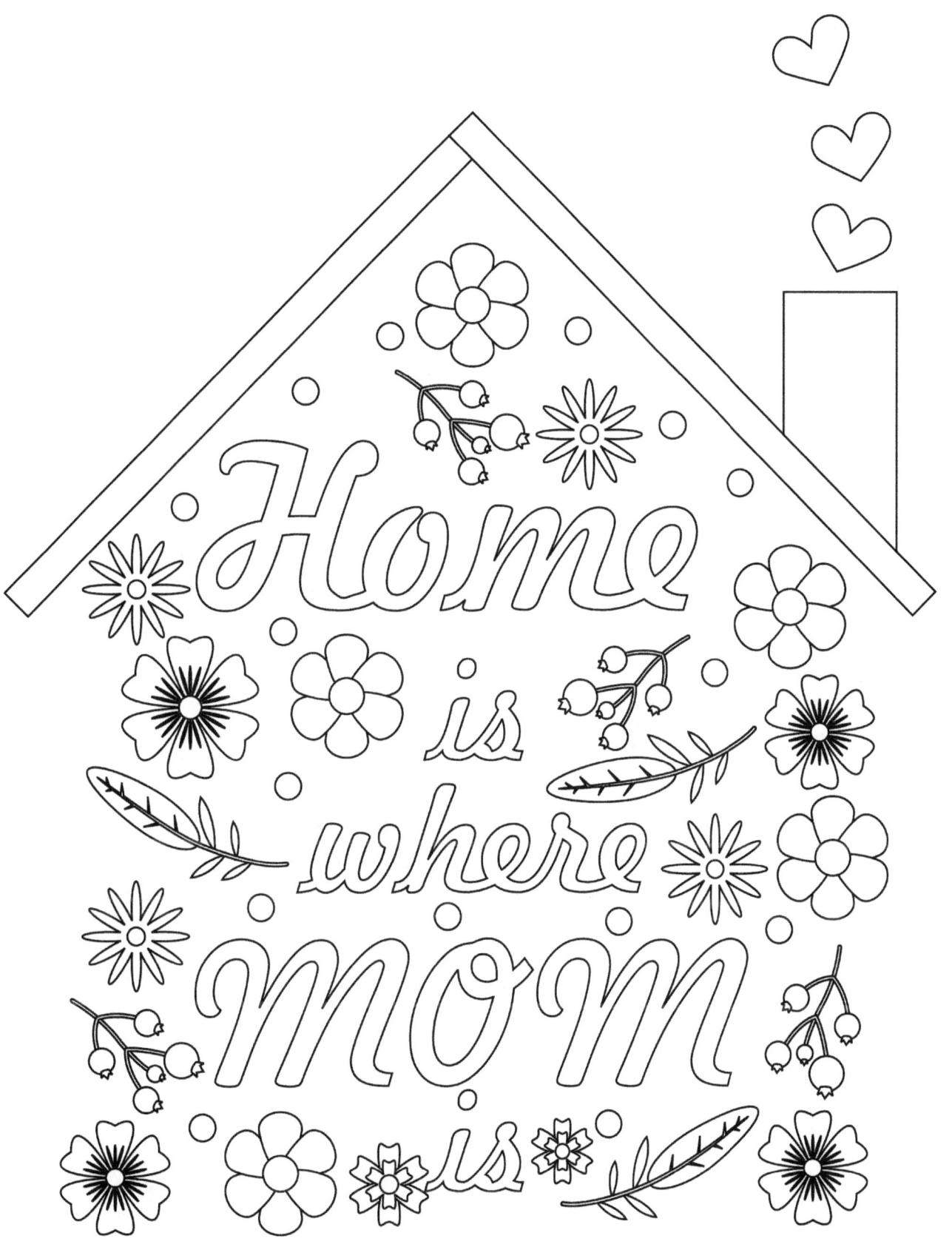

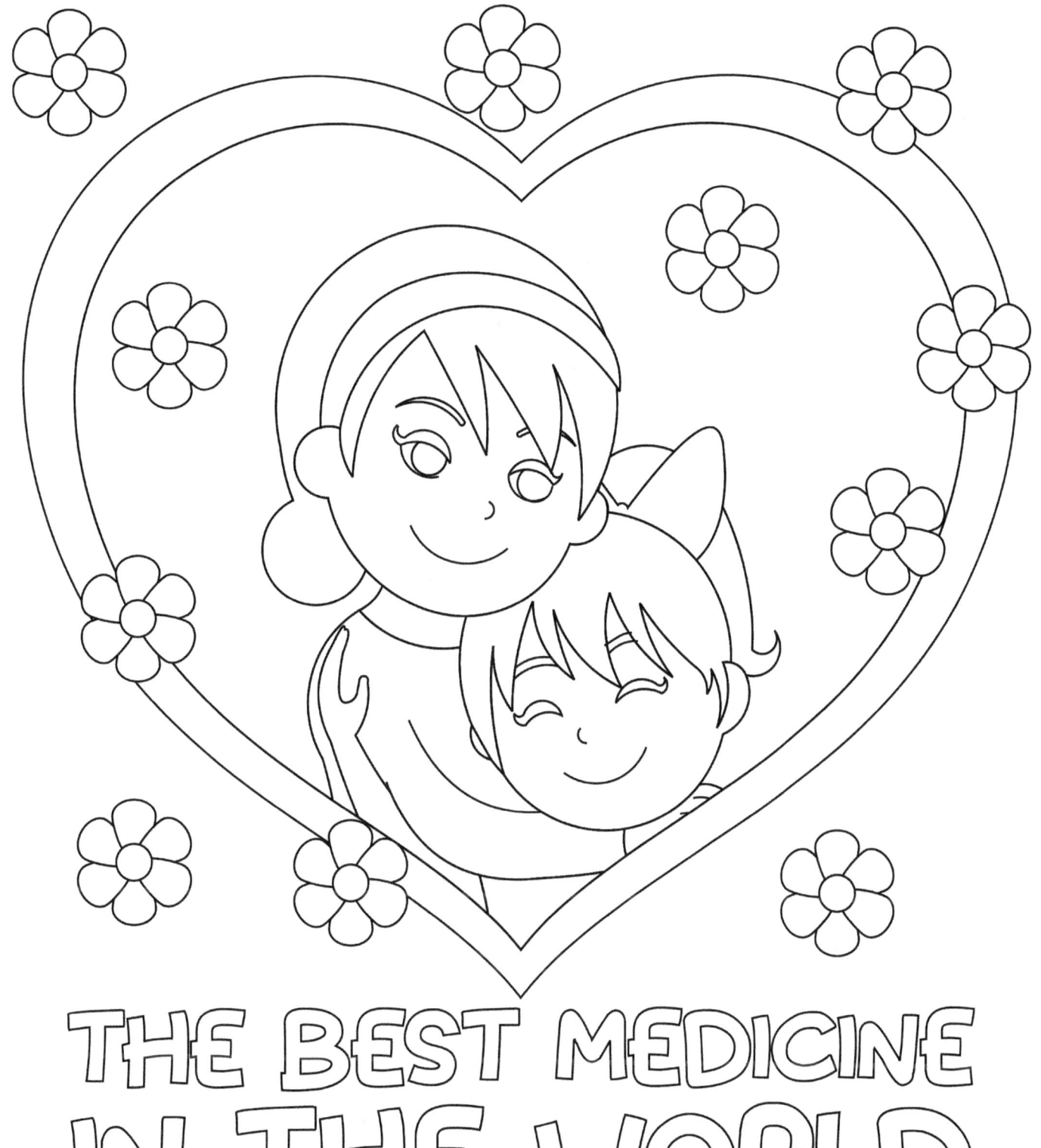

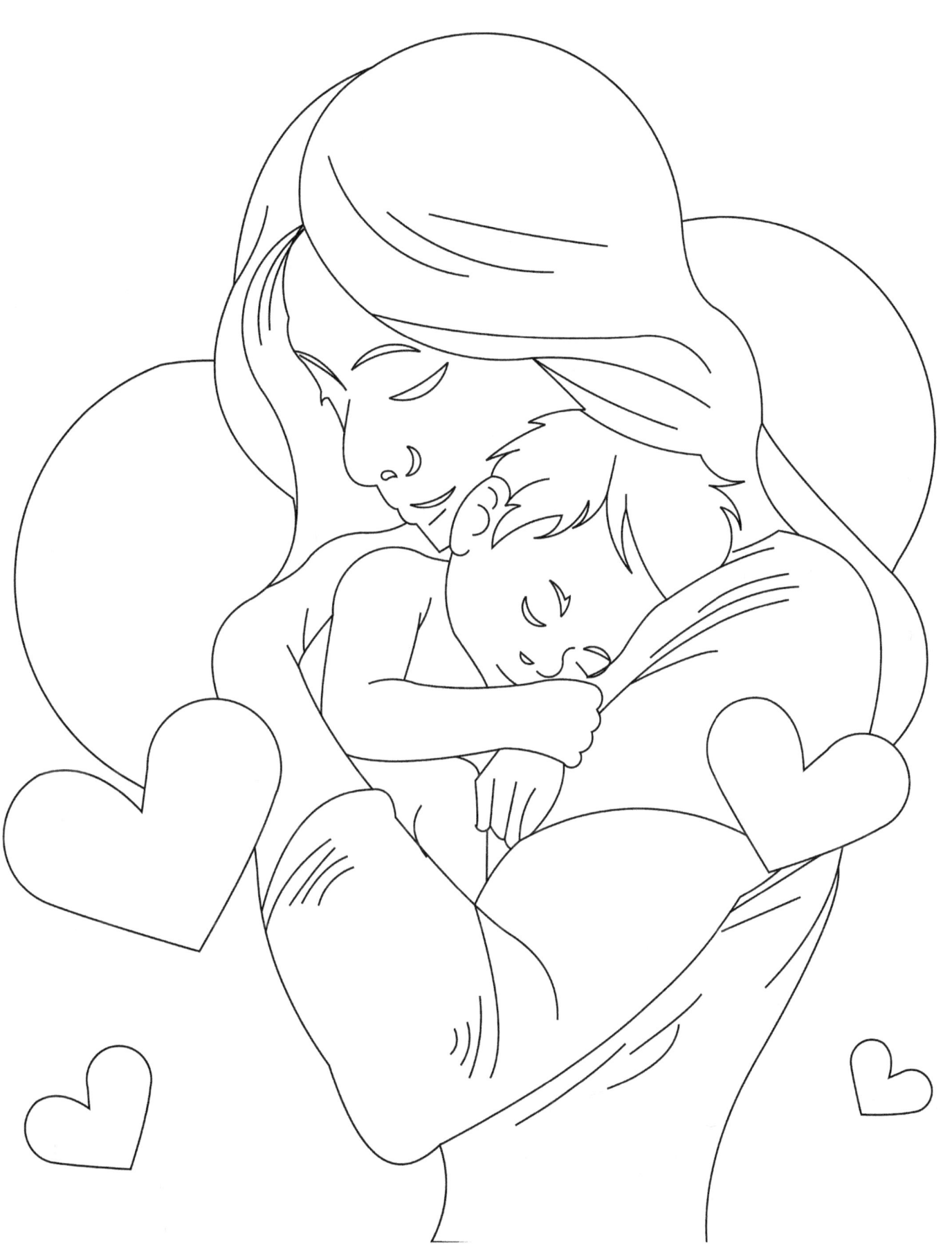

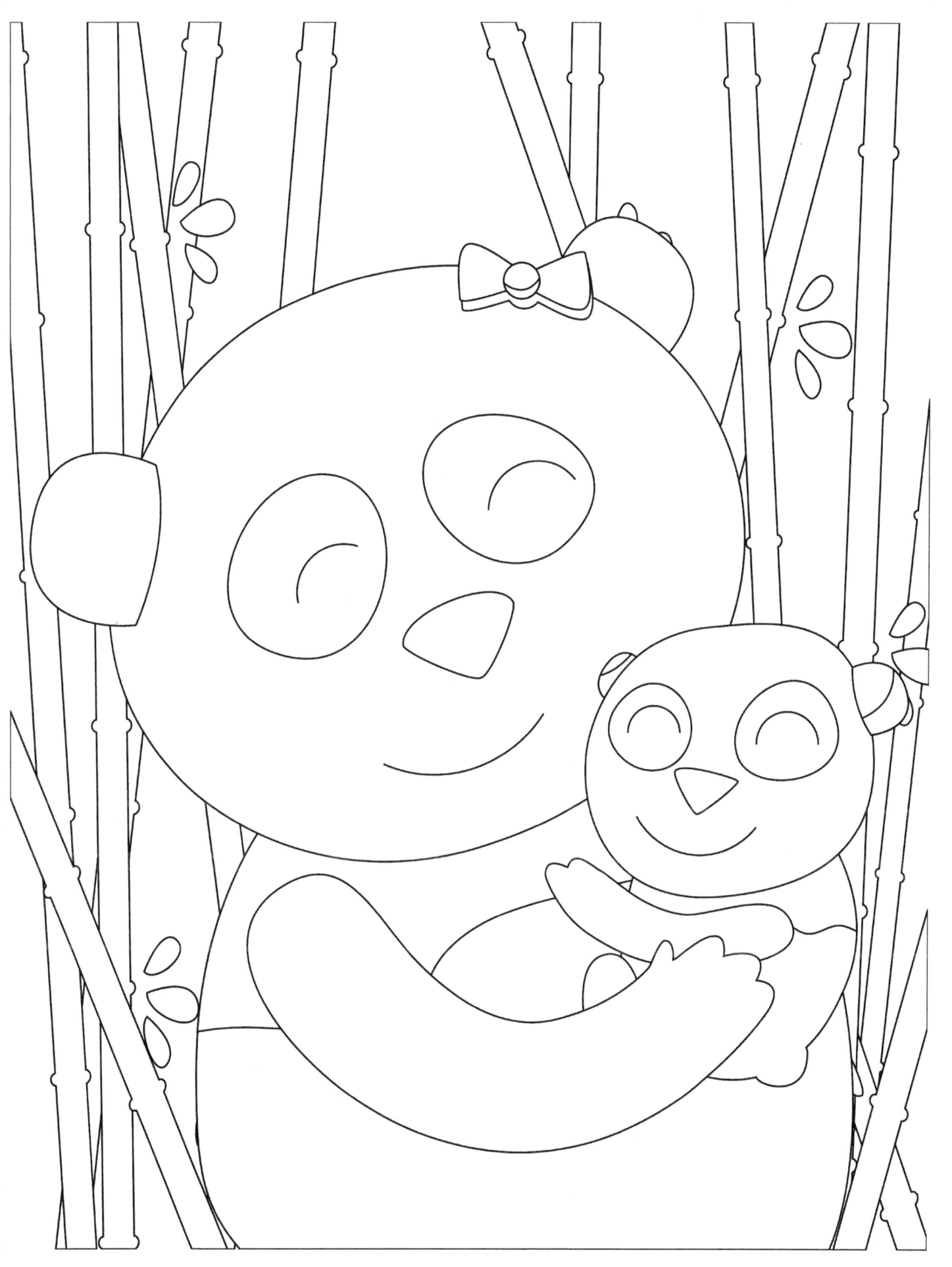

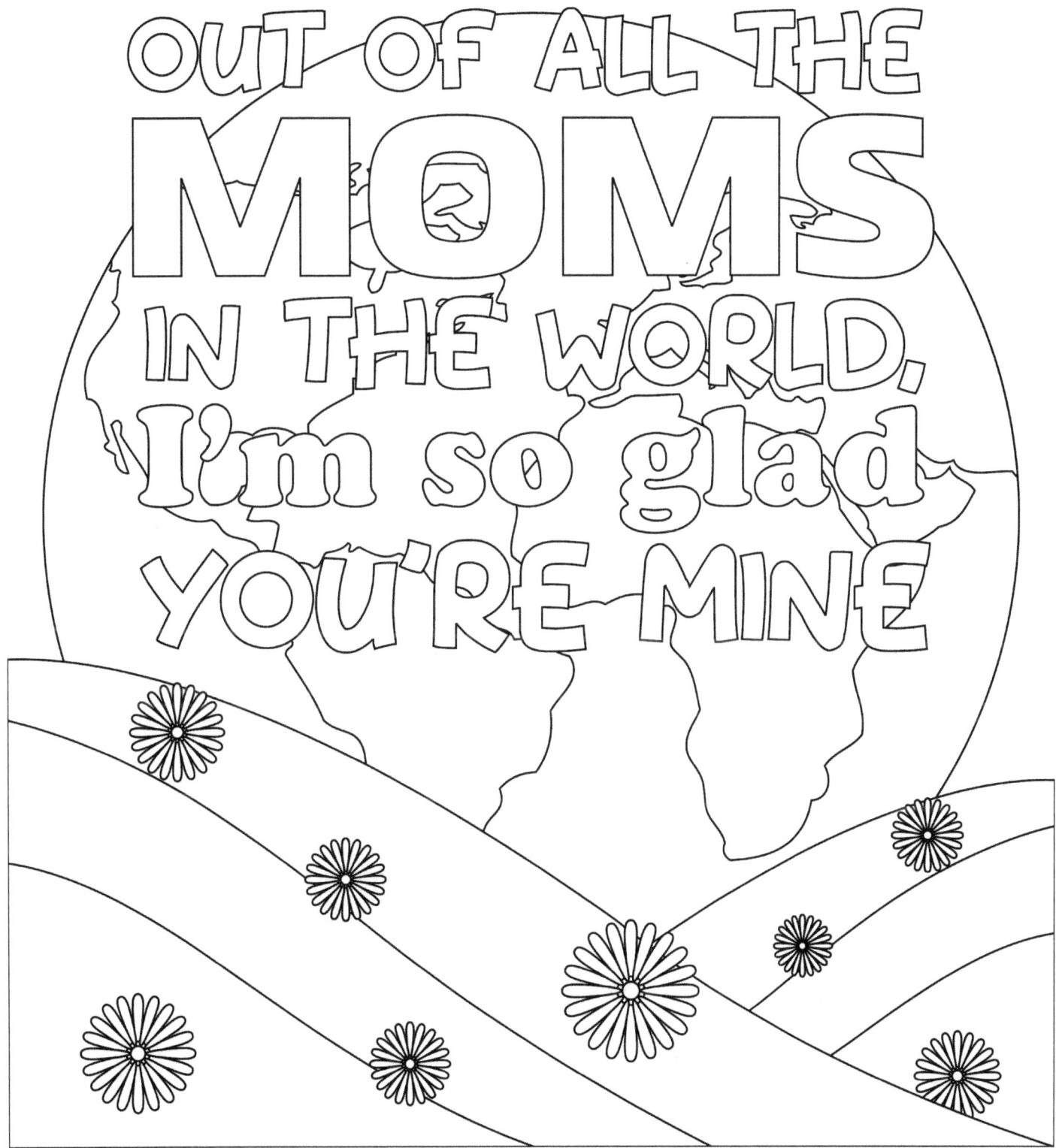

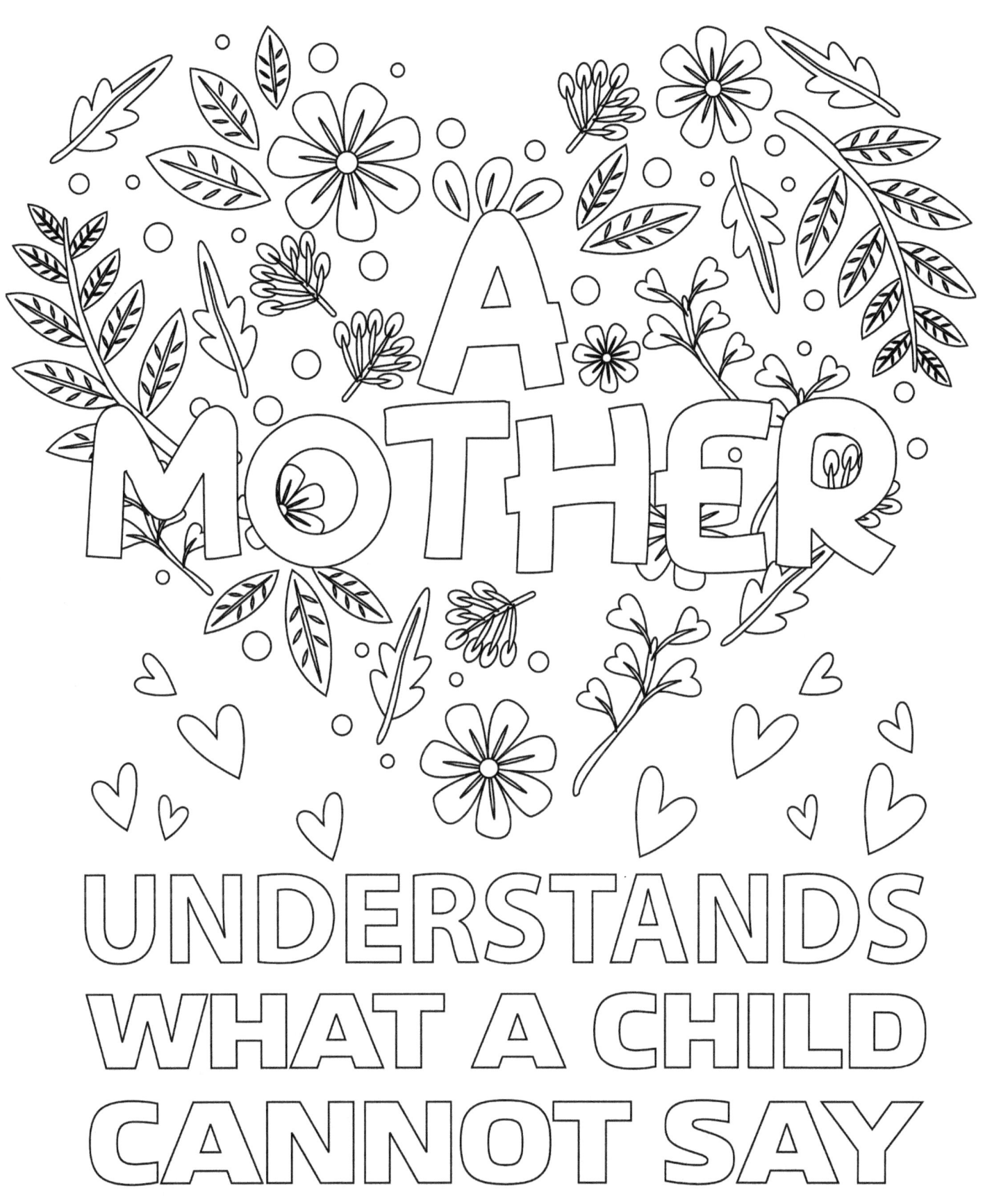

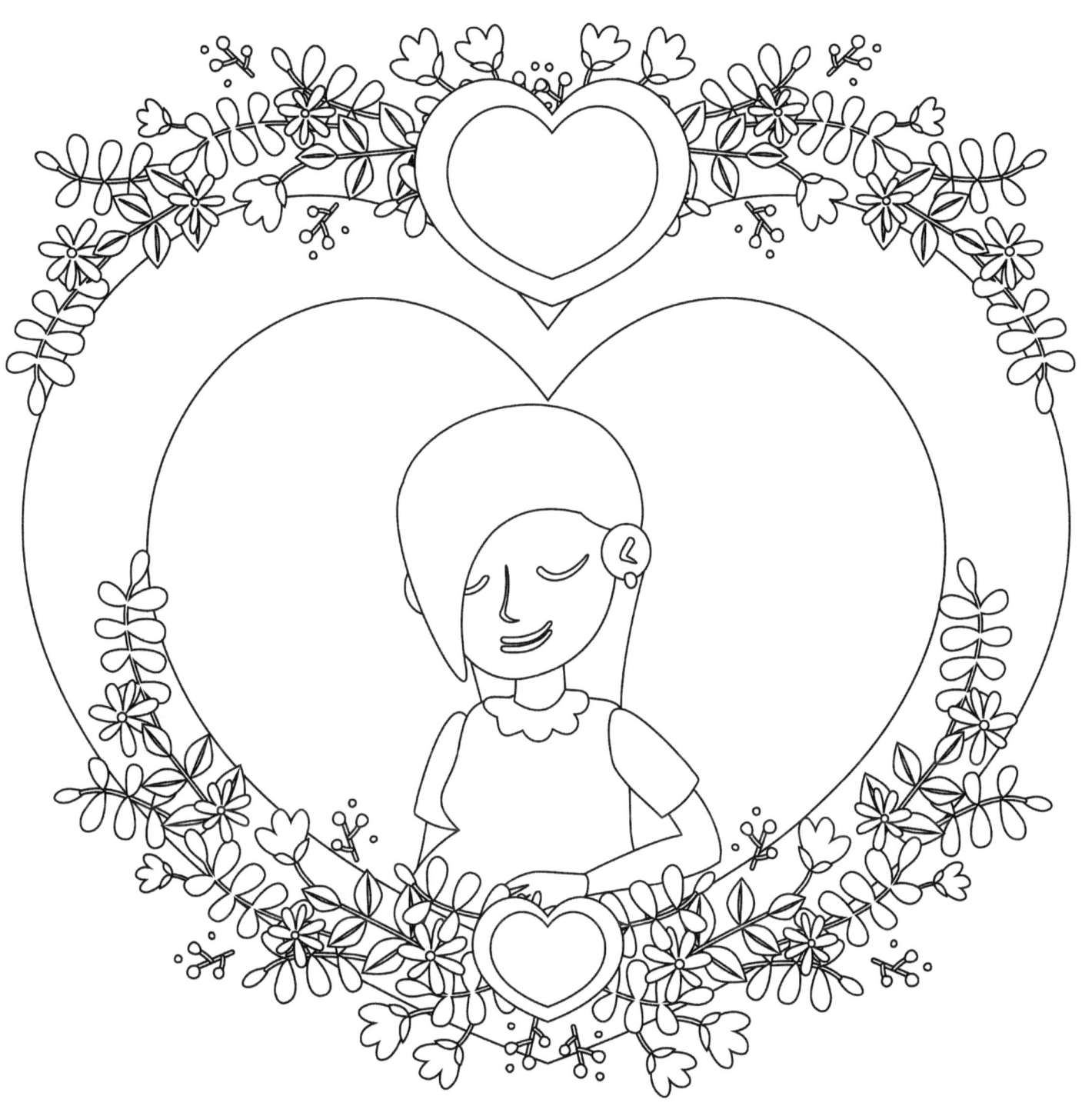

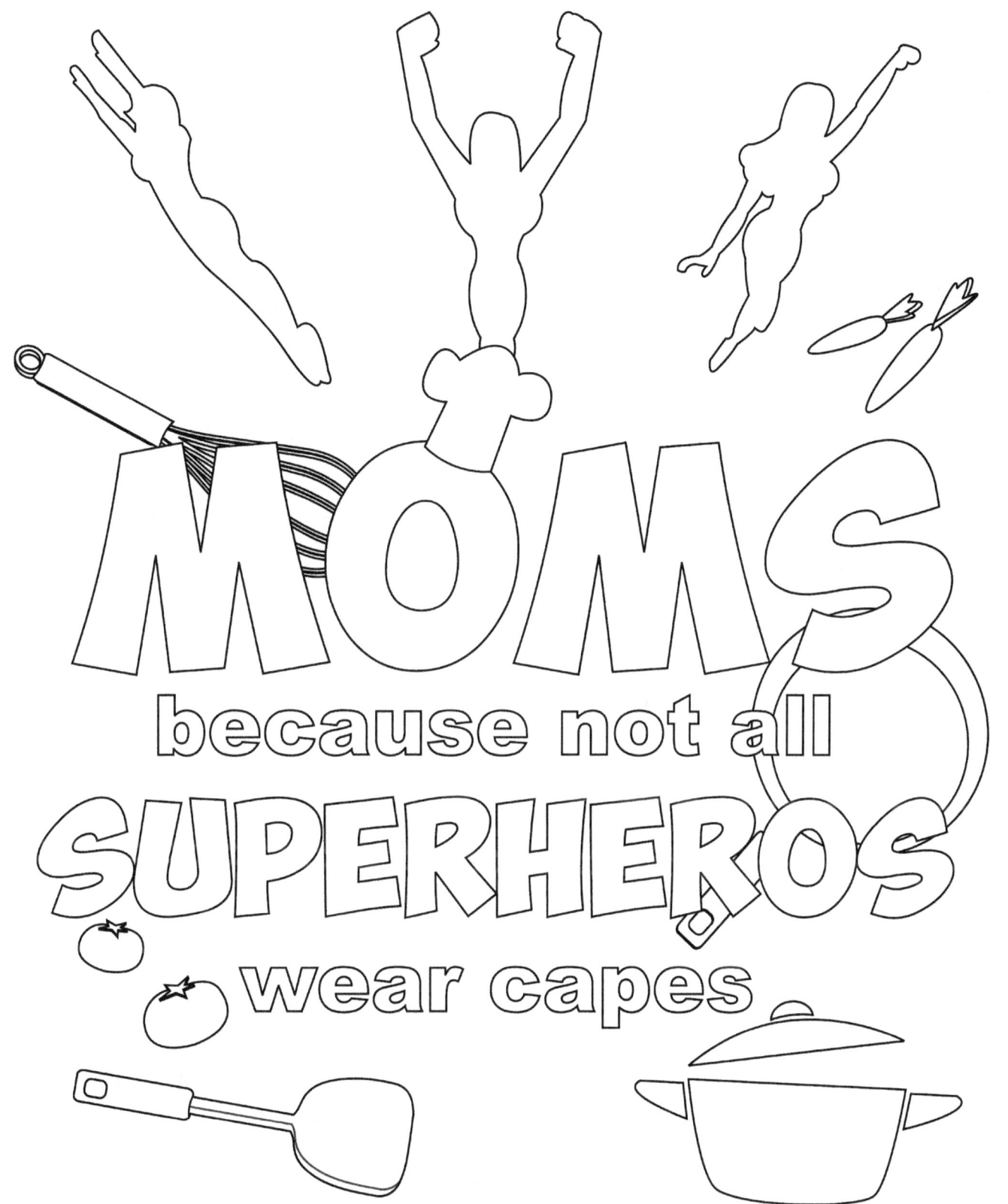

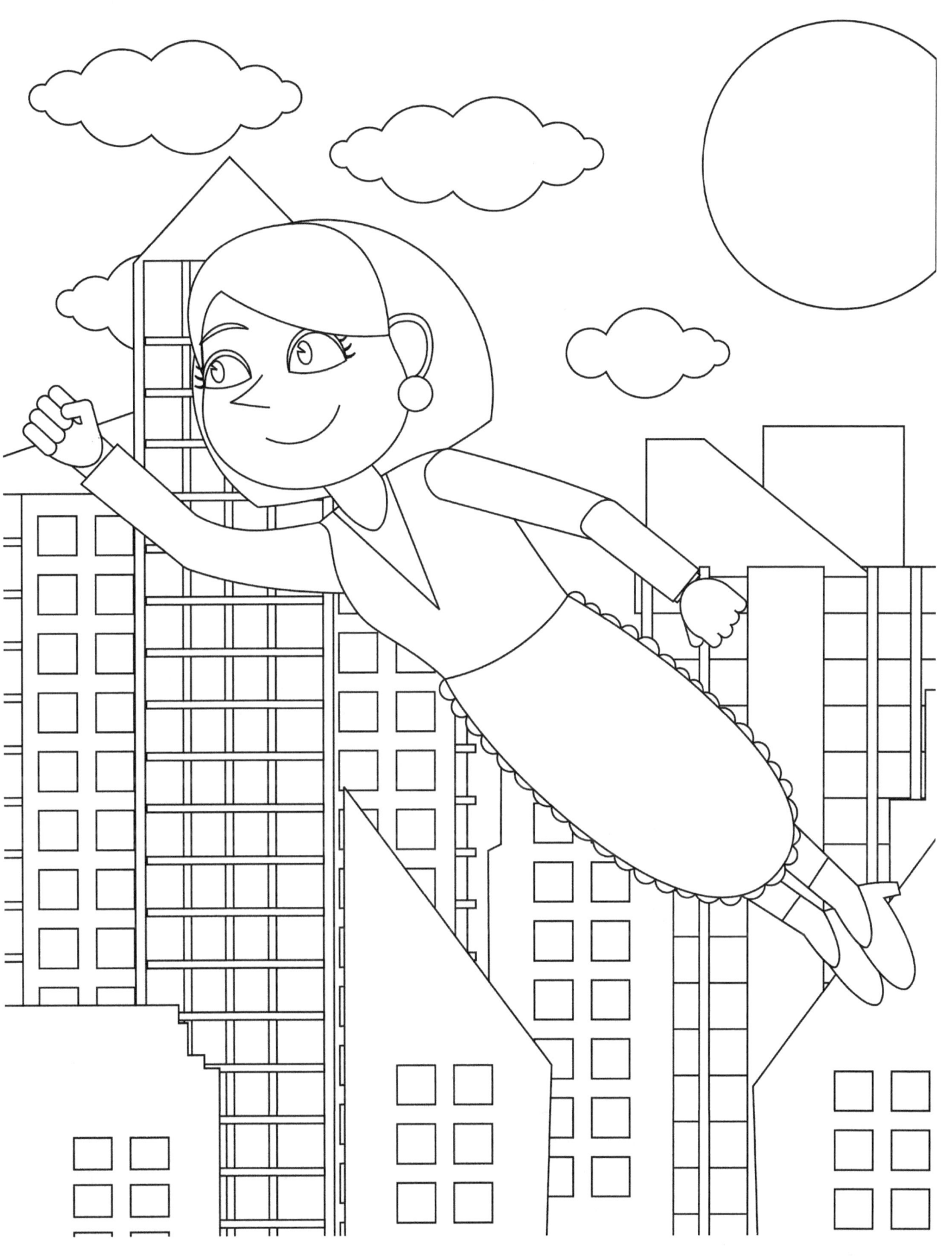

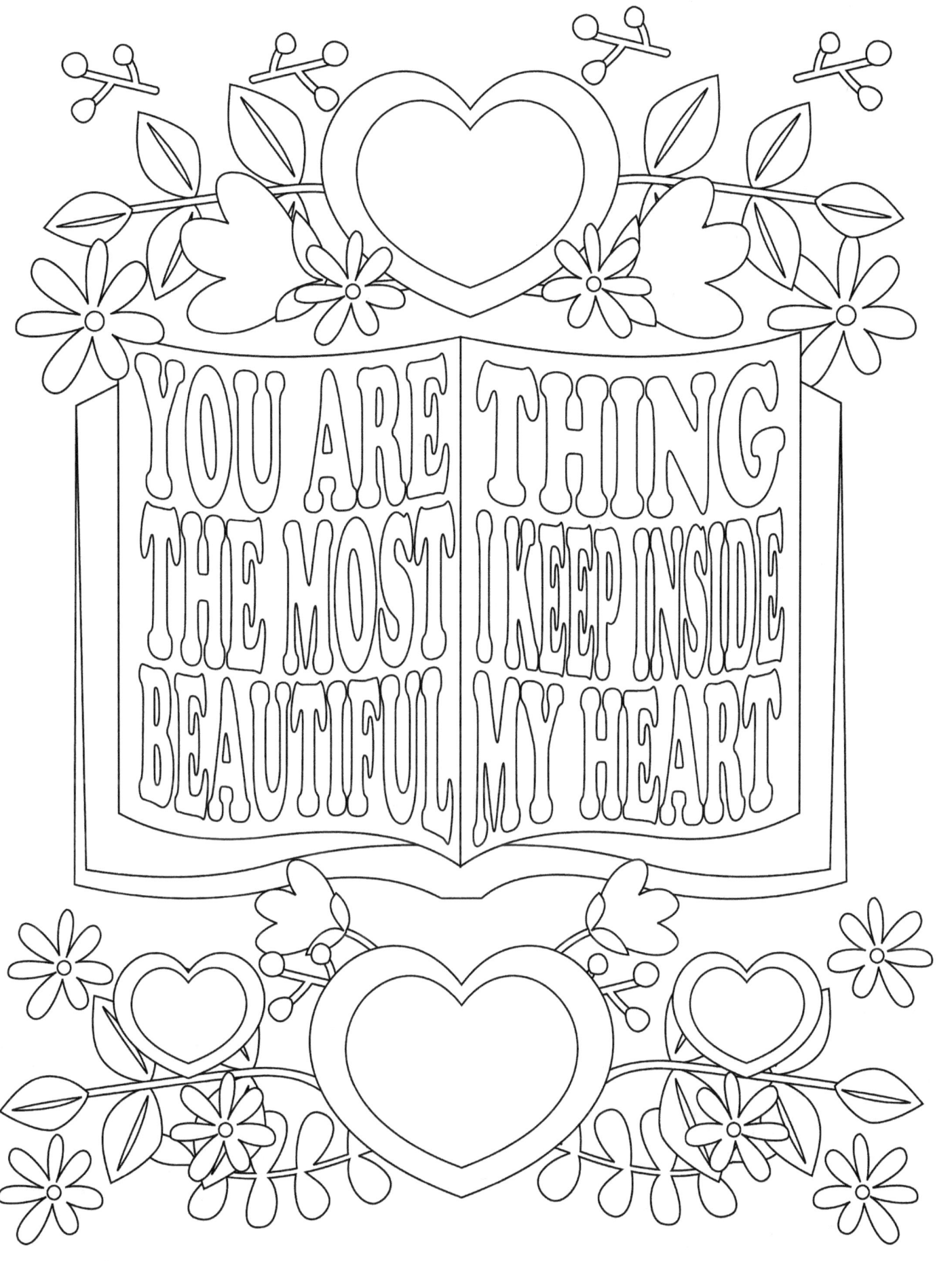

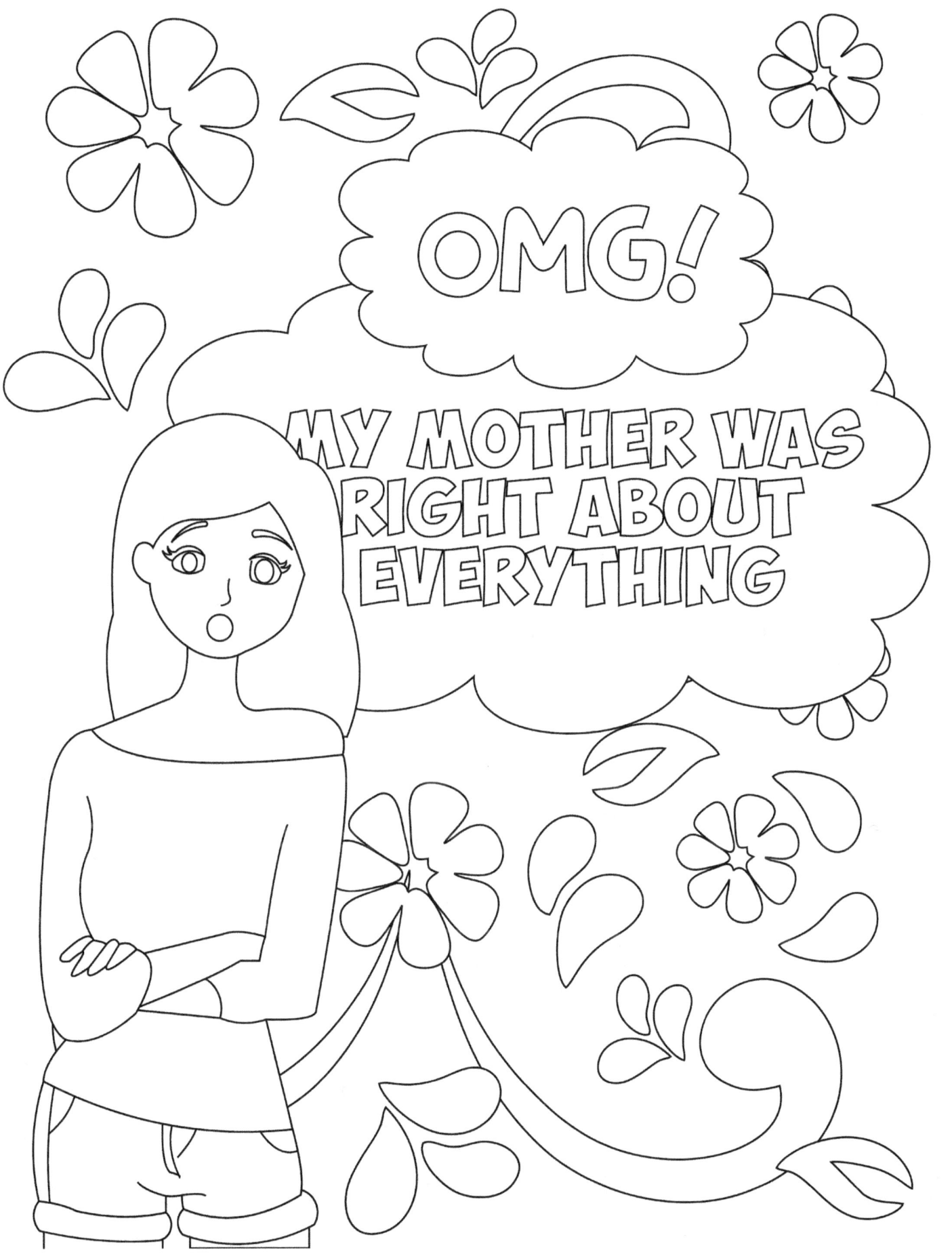

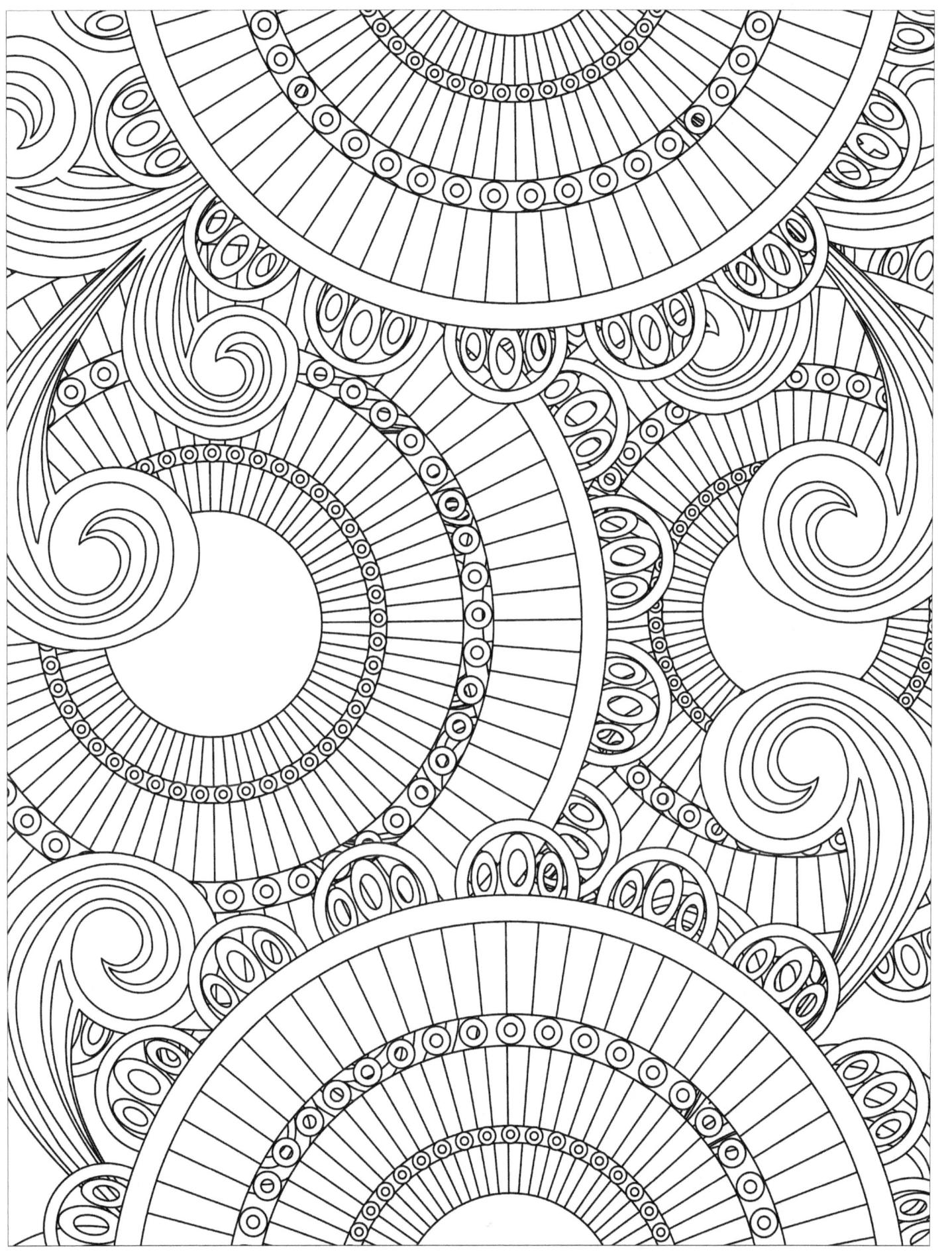

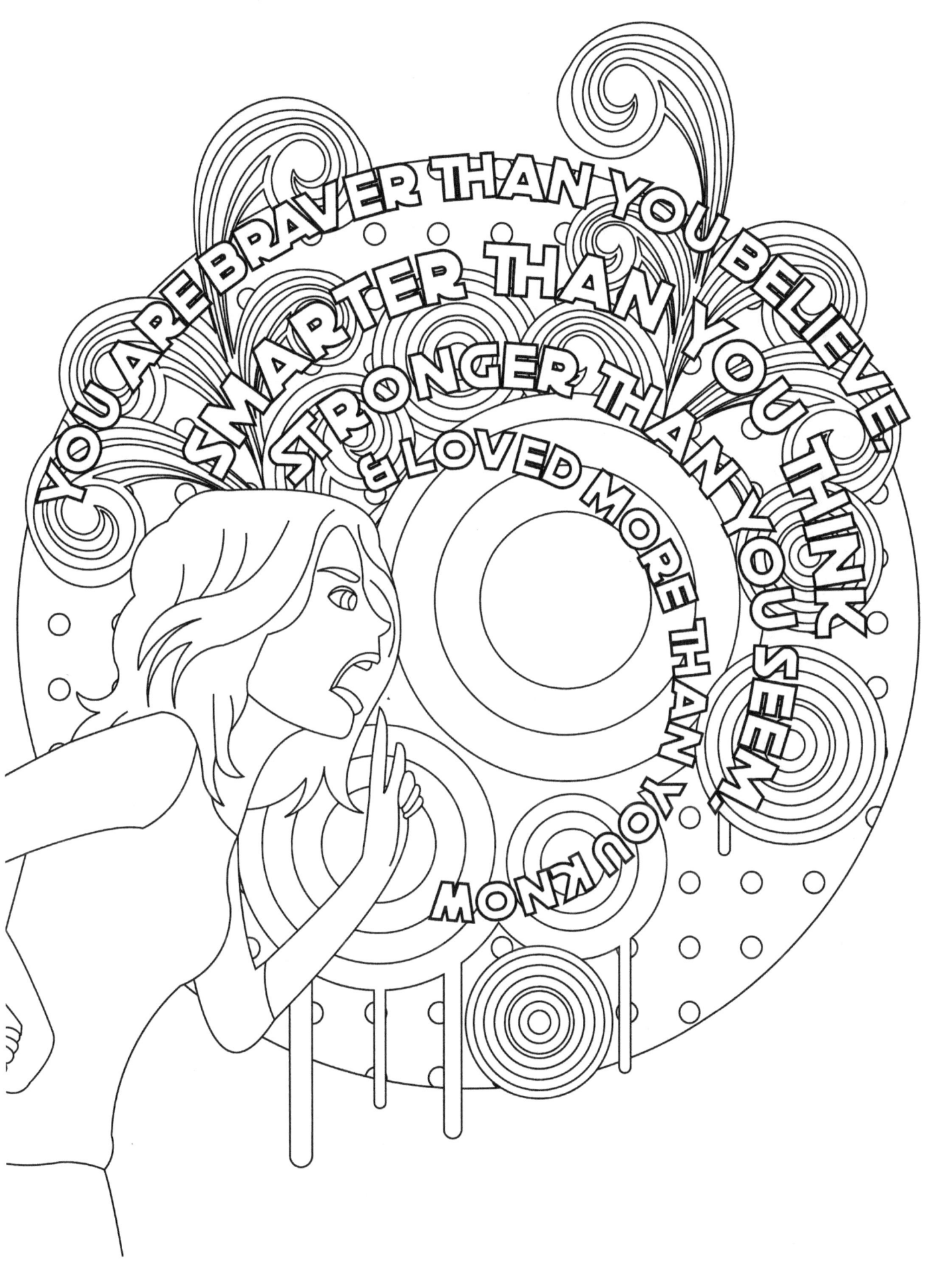

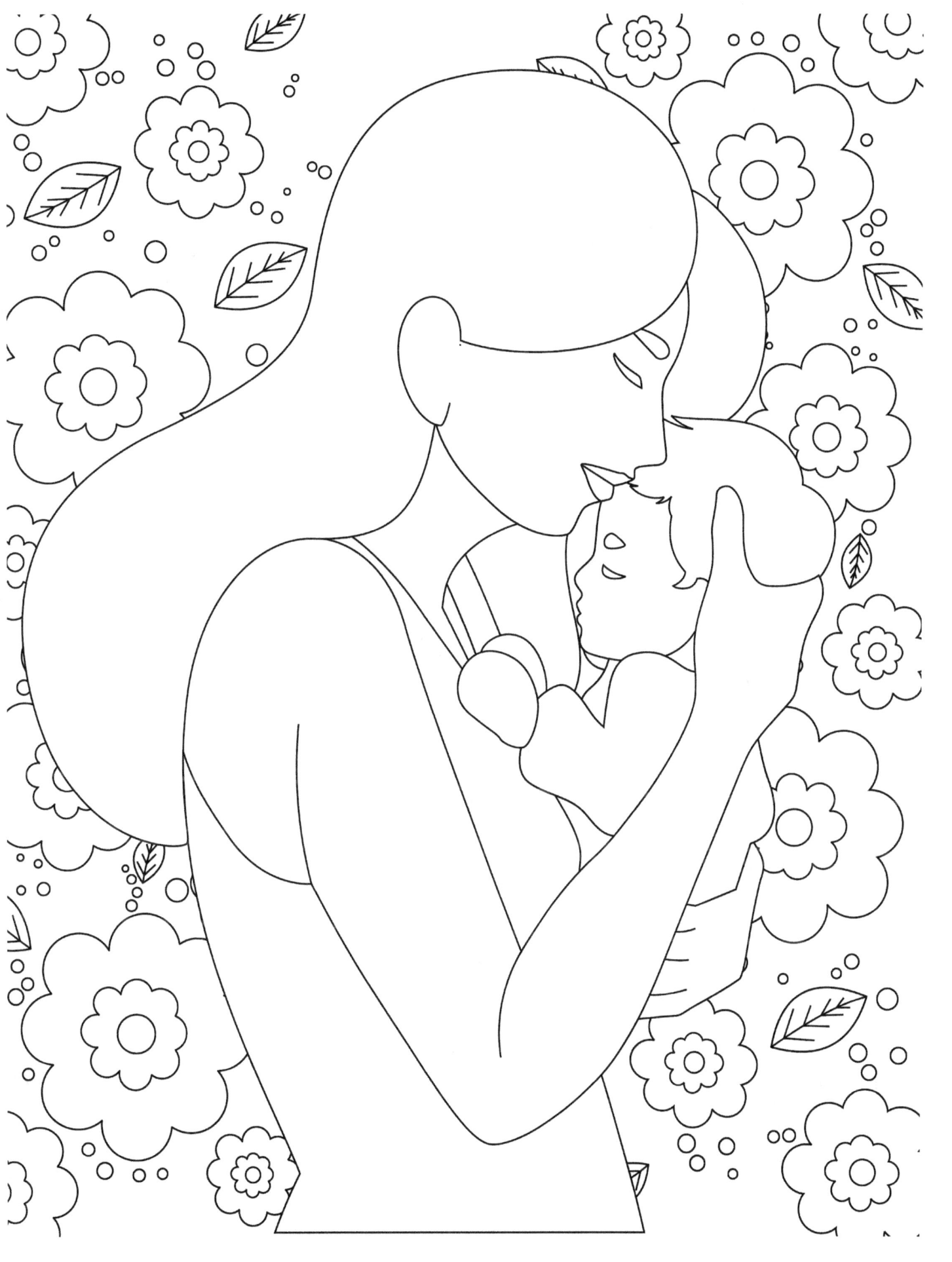

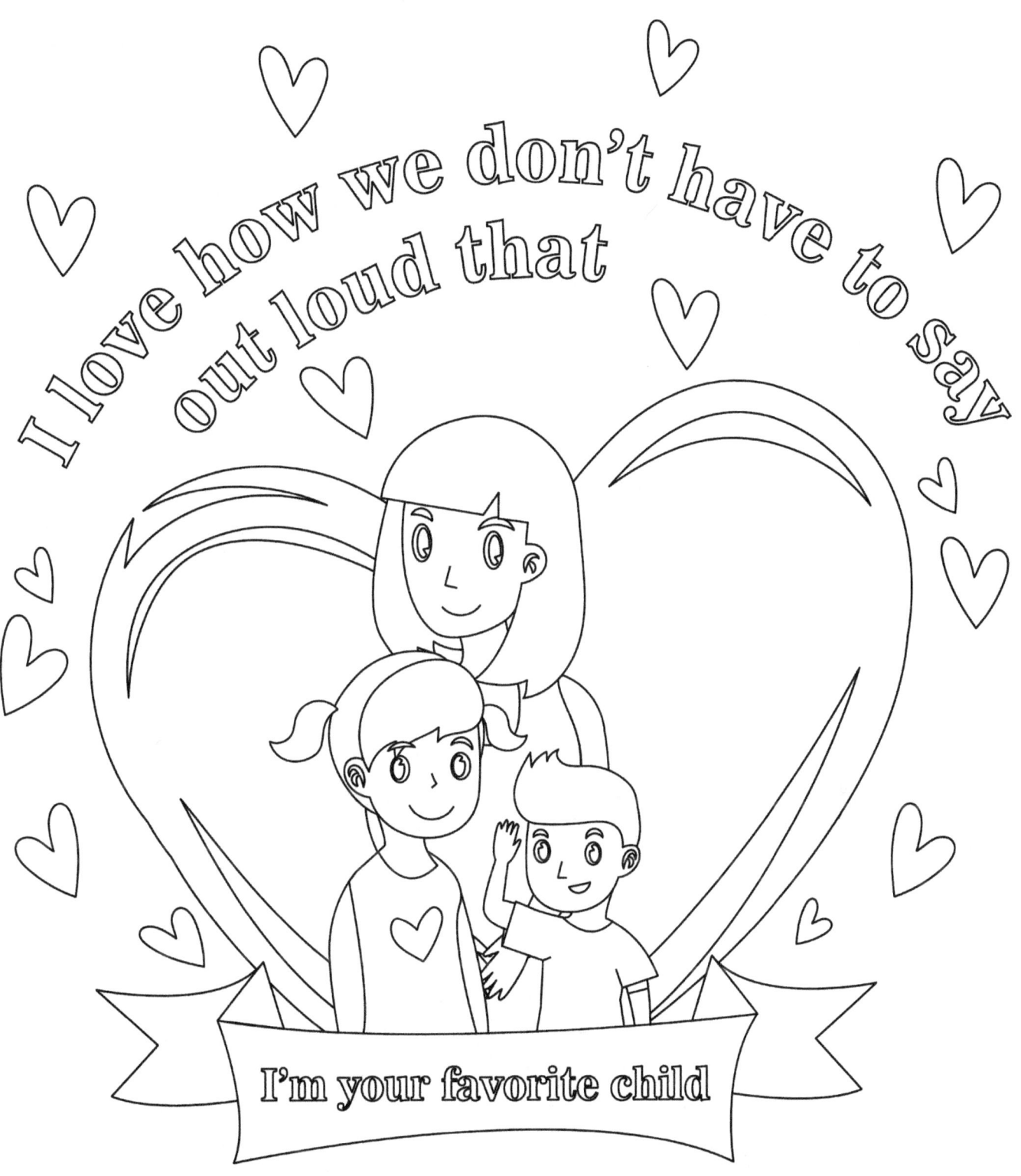

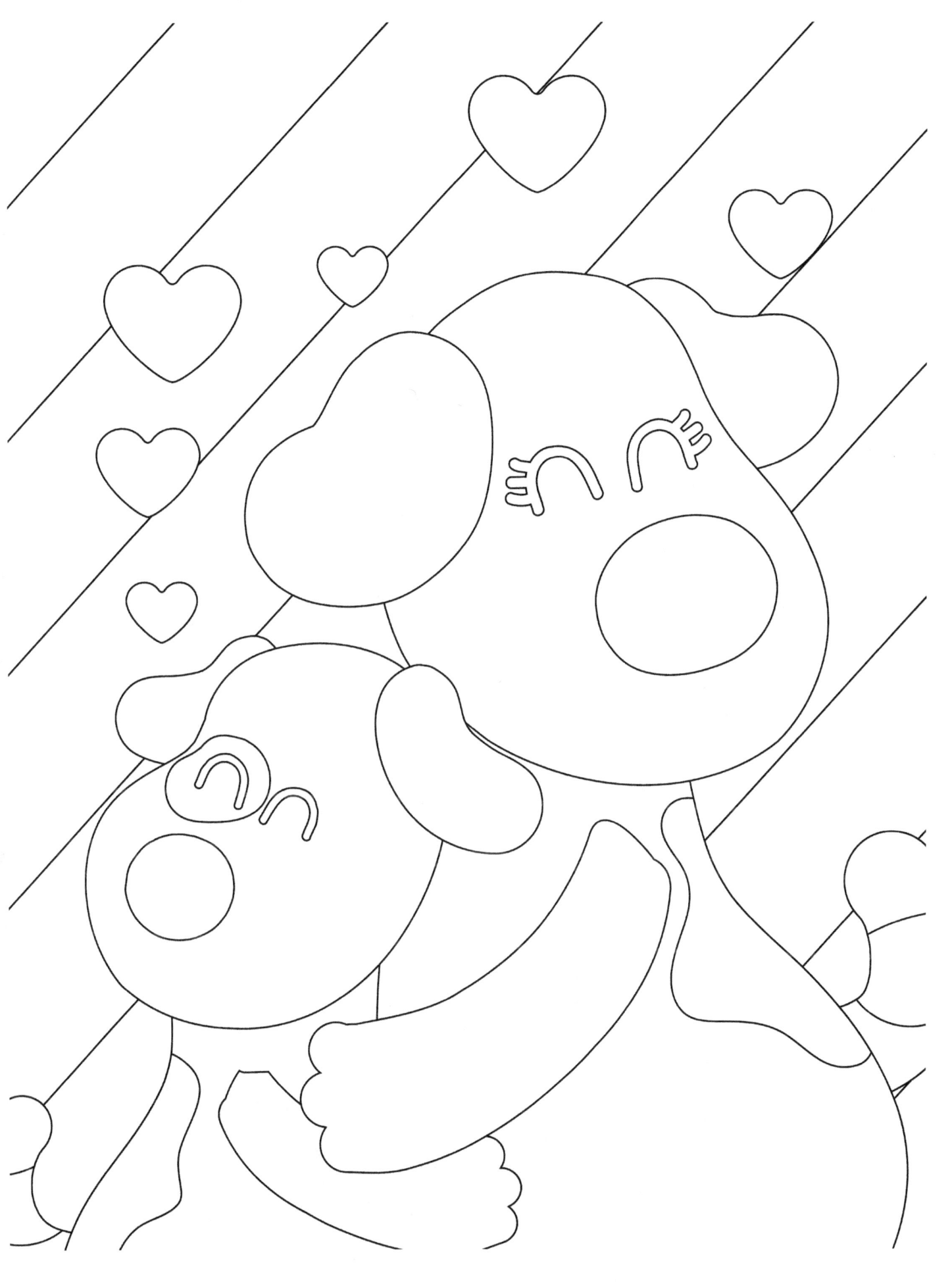

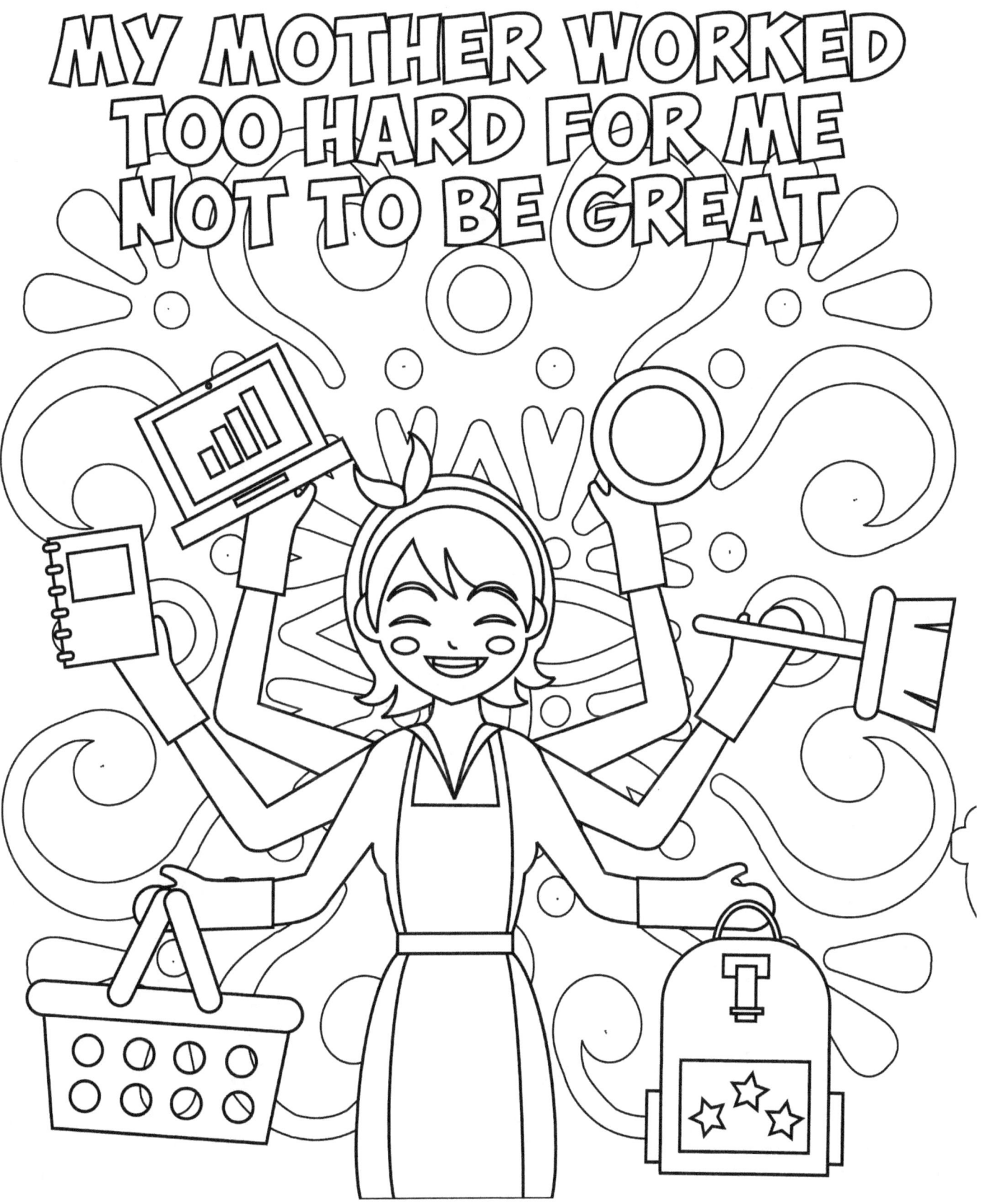

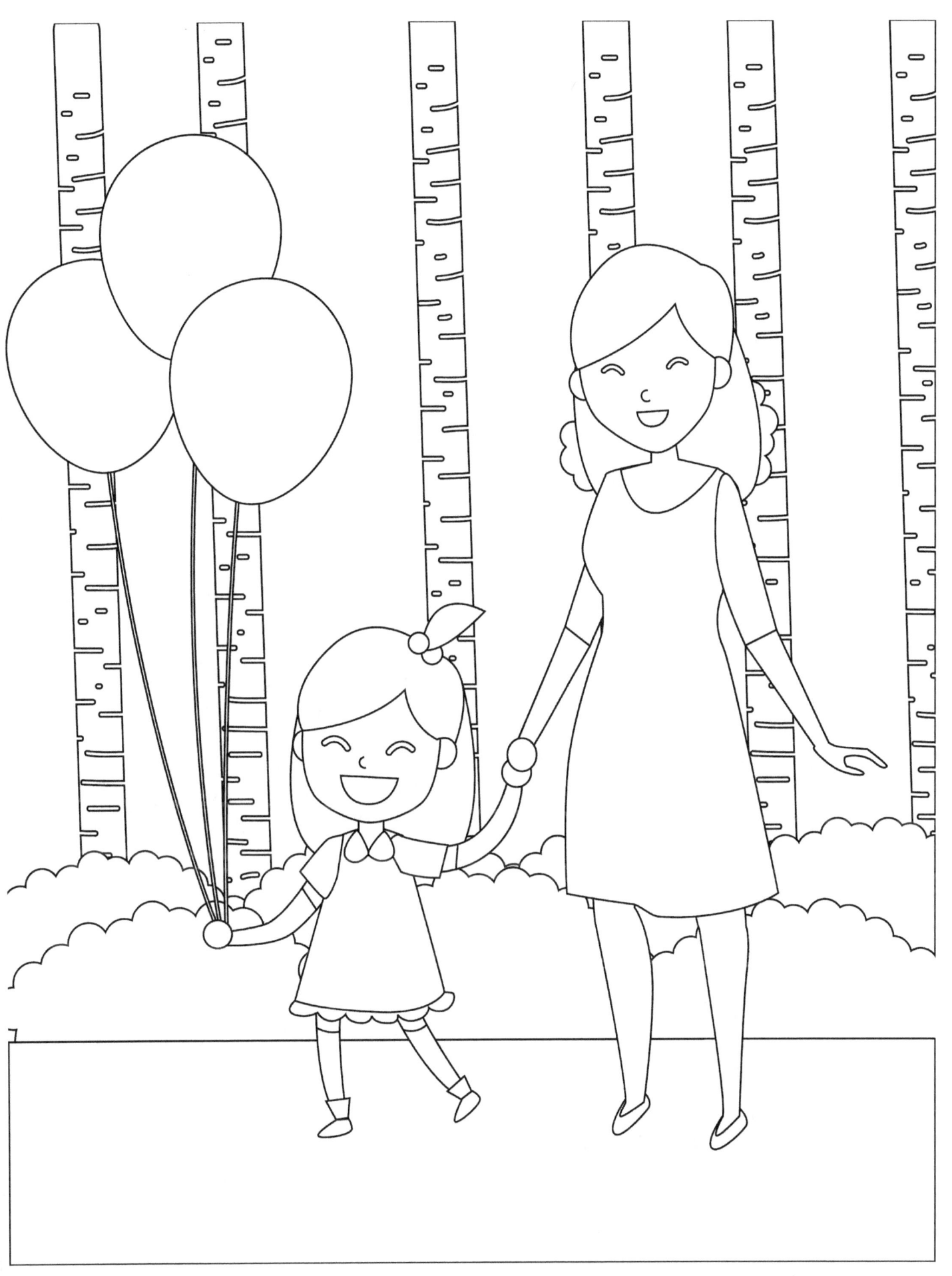

BONUS

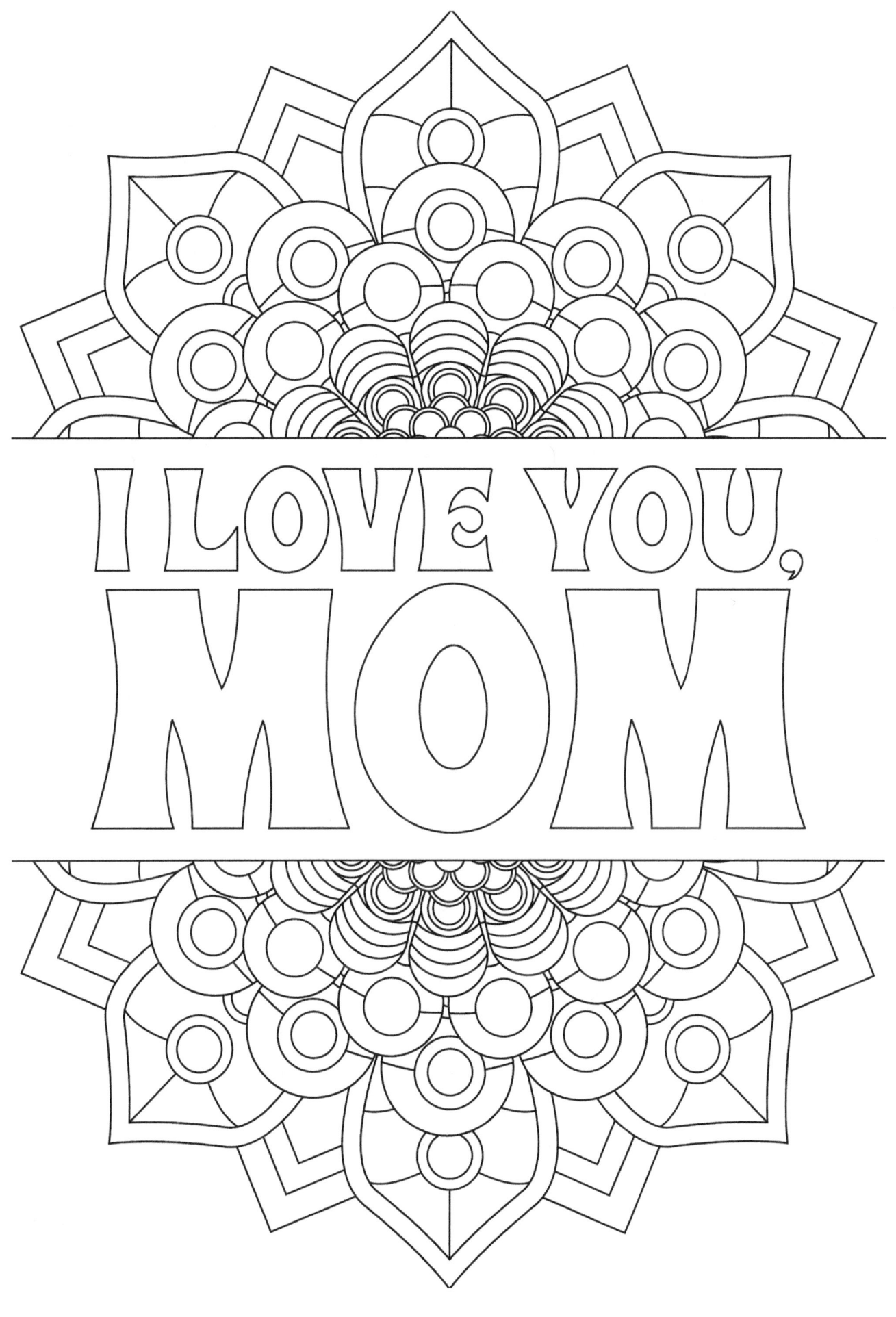

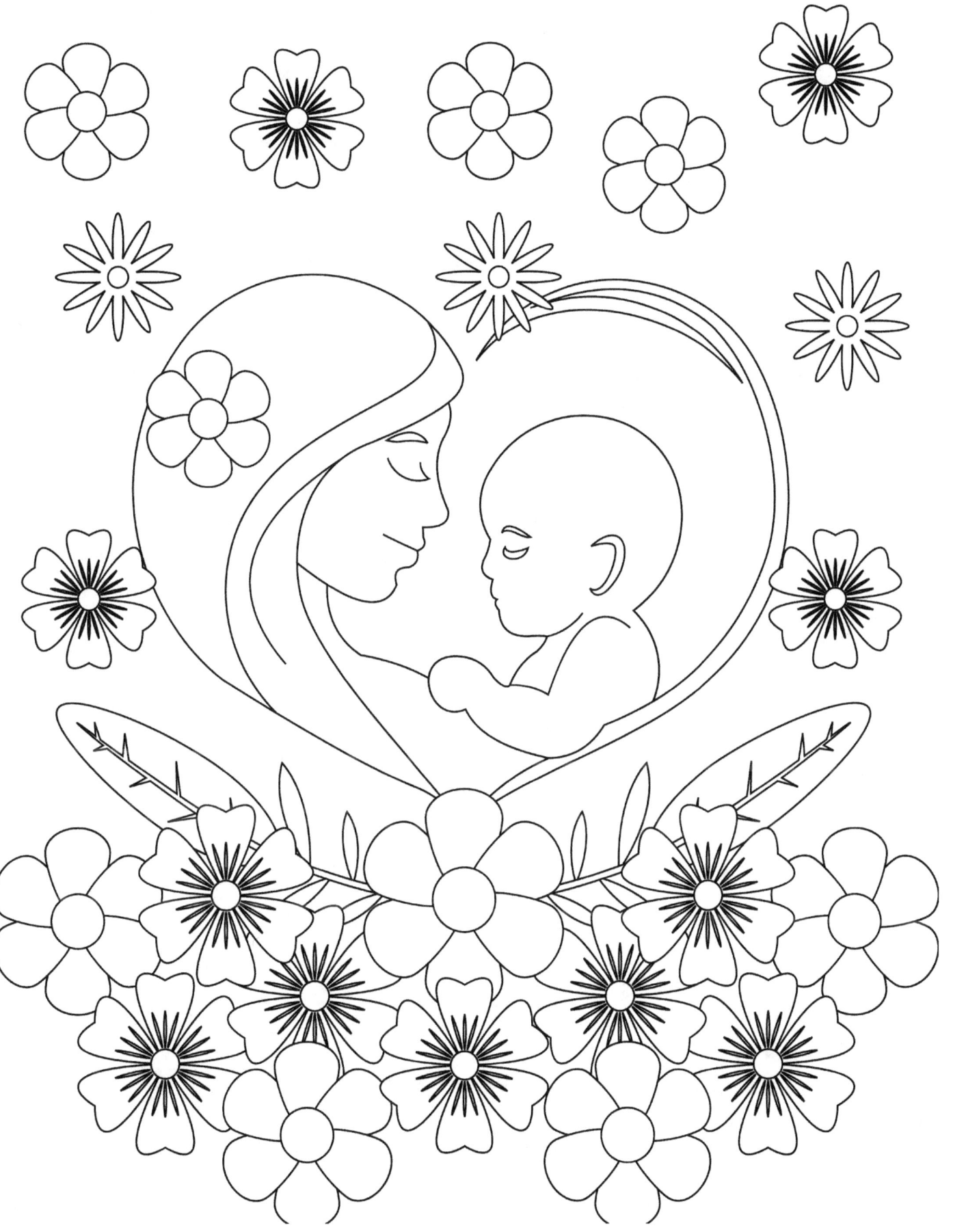

Life doesn't come with a manual,

IT COMES WITH A MOTHER

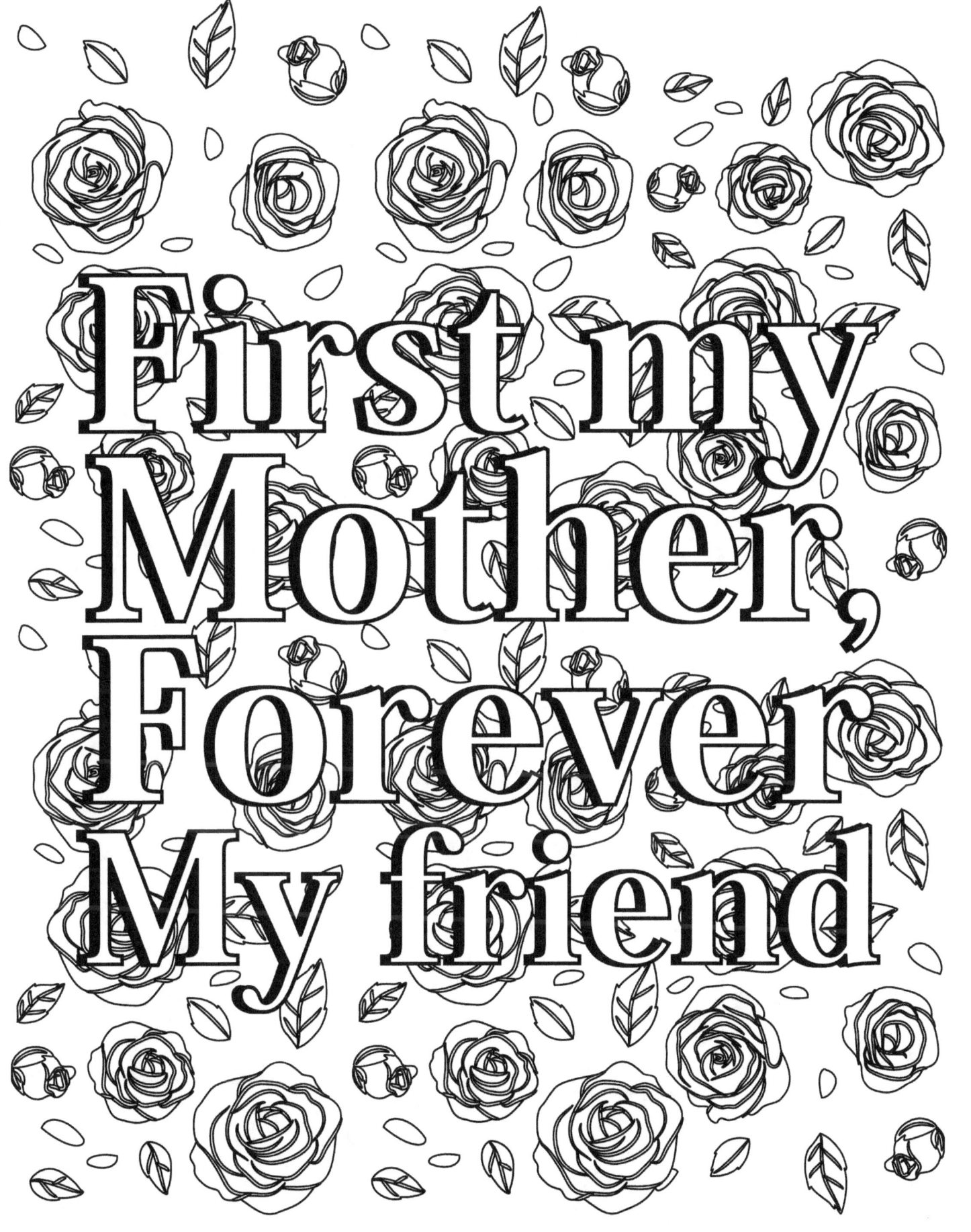

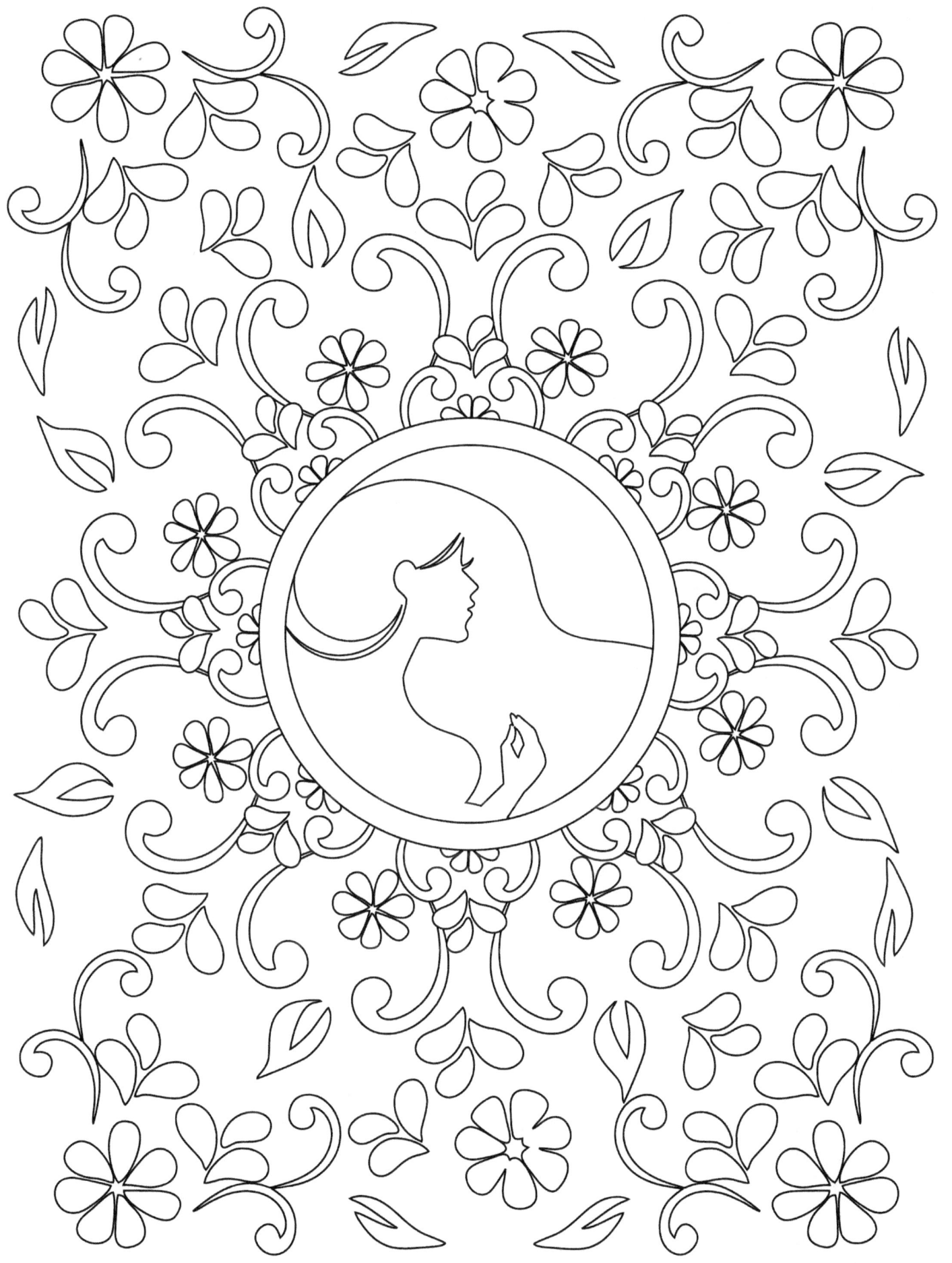

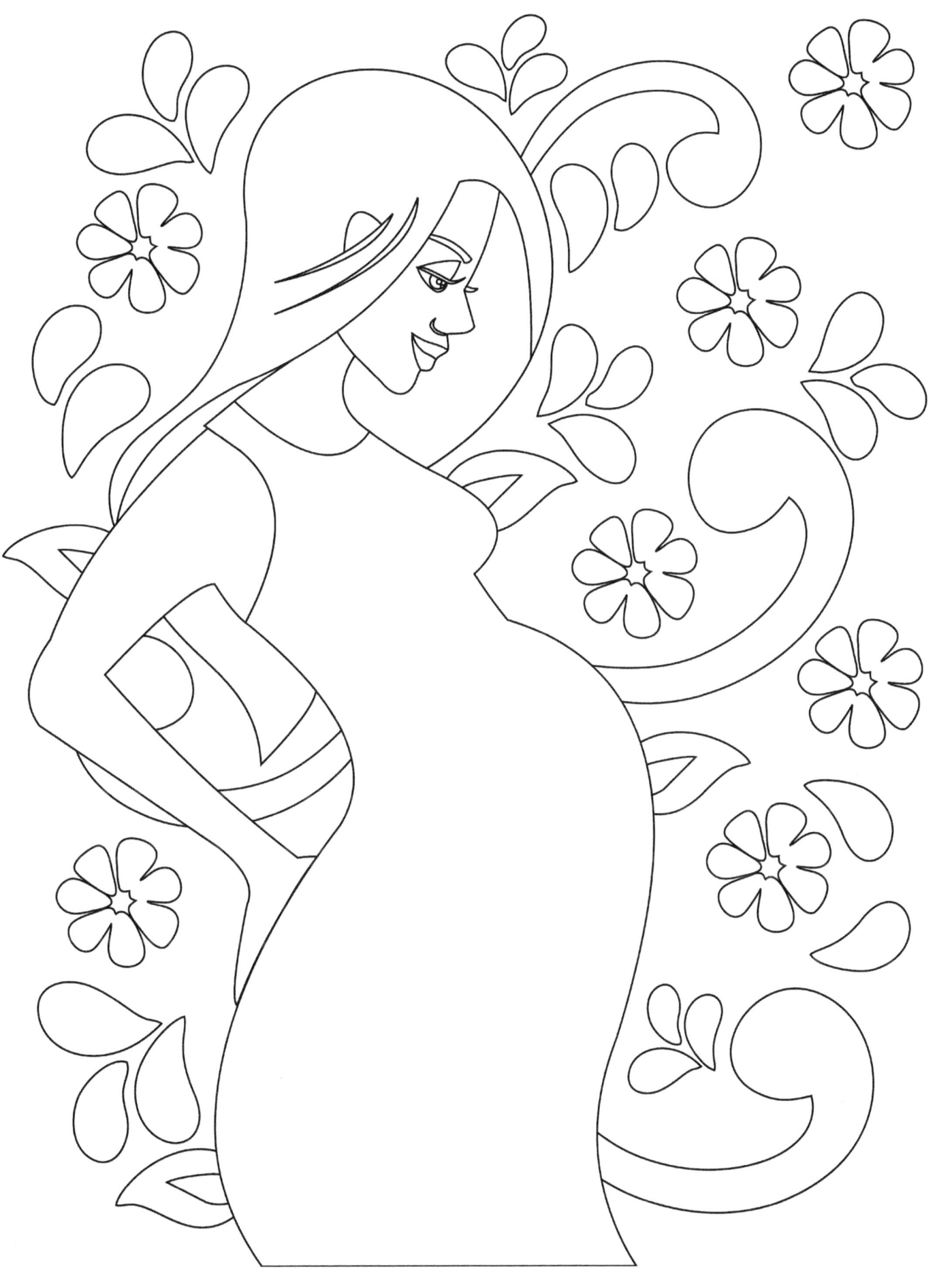

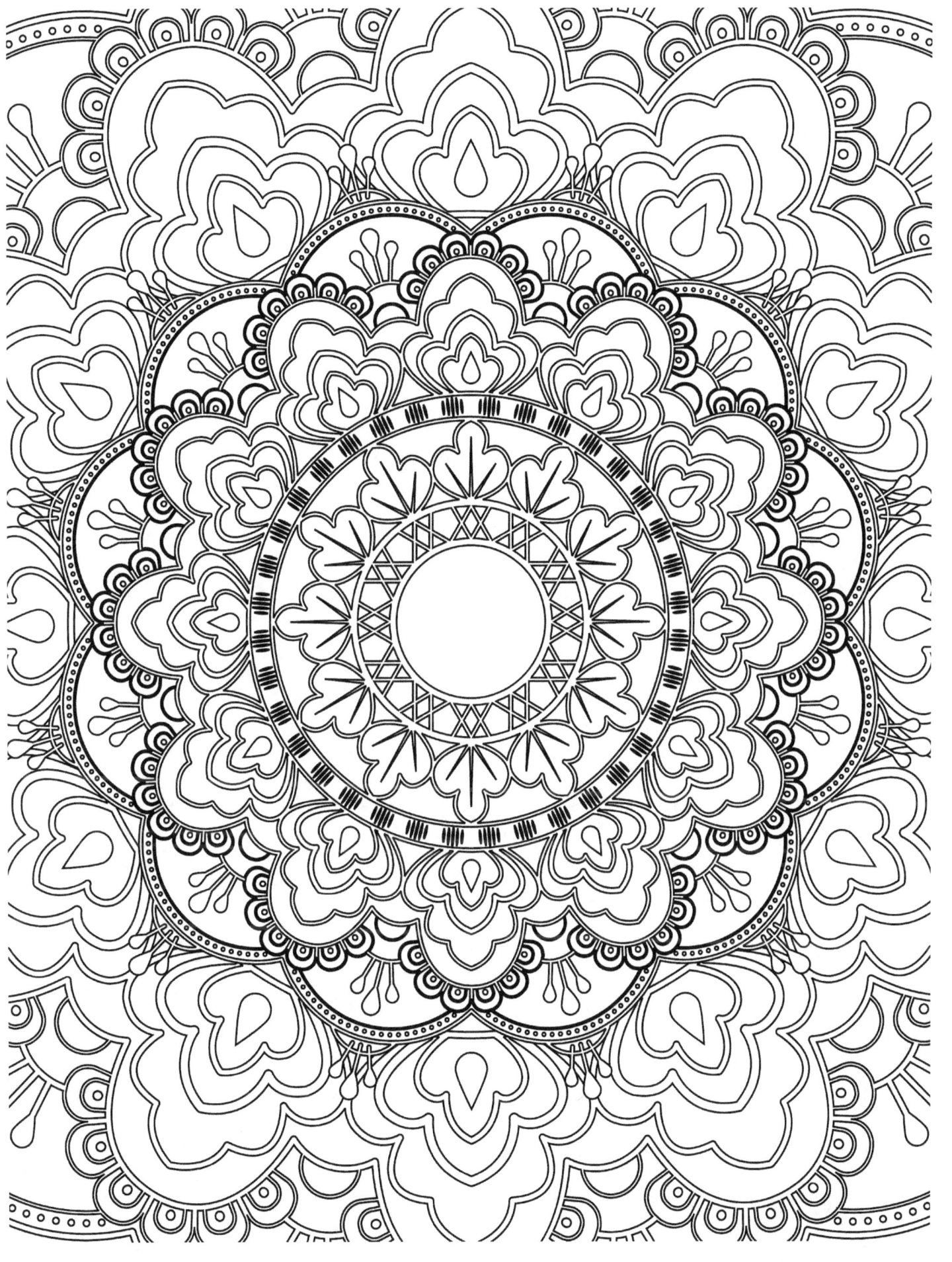

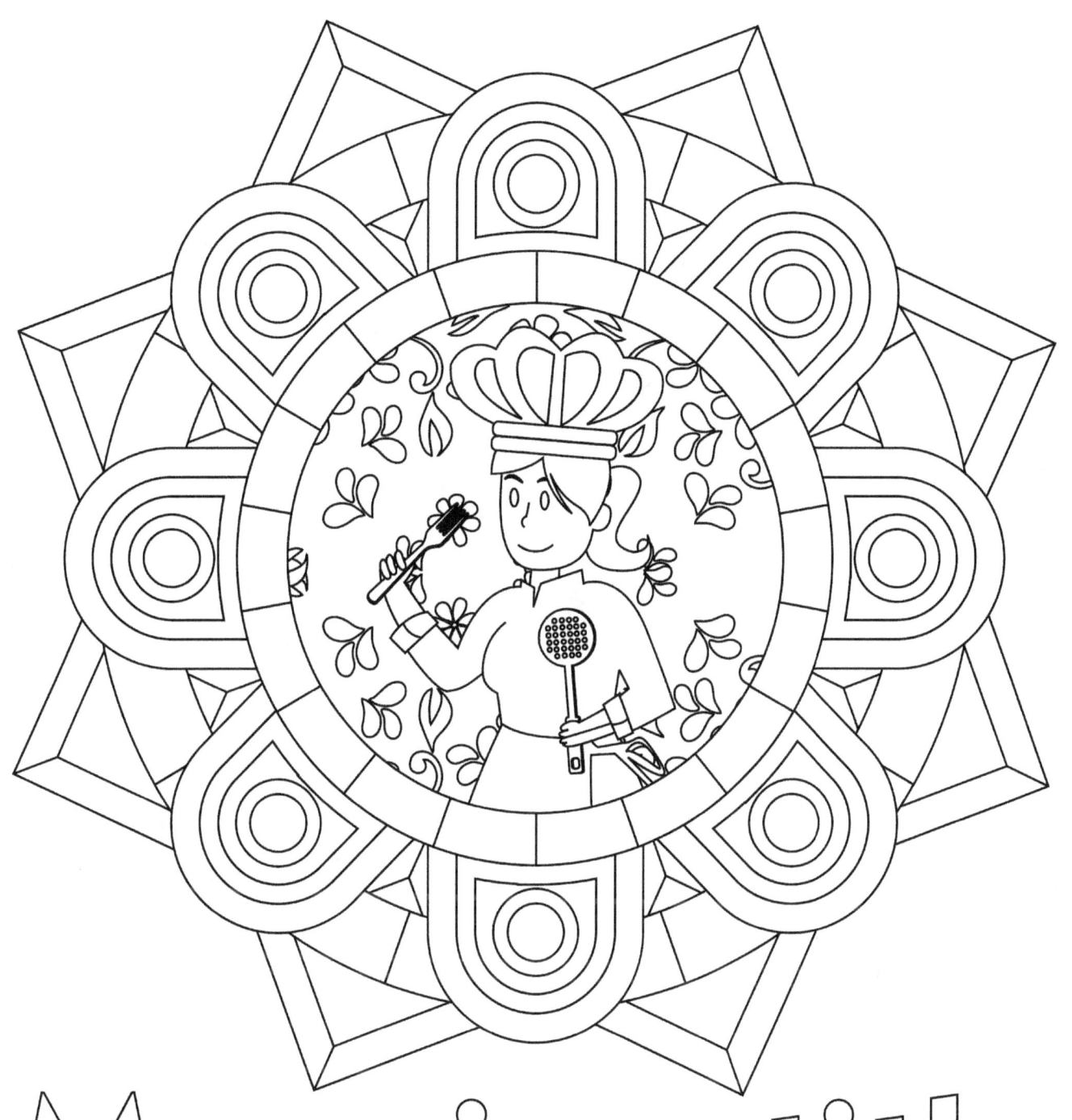

Mom is a title just above Queen

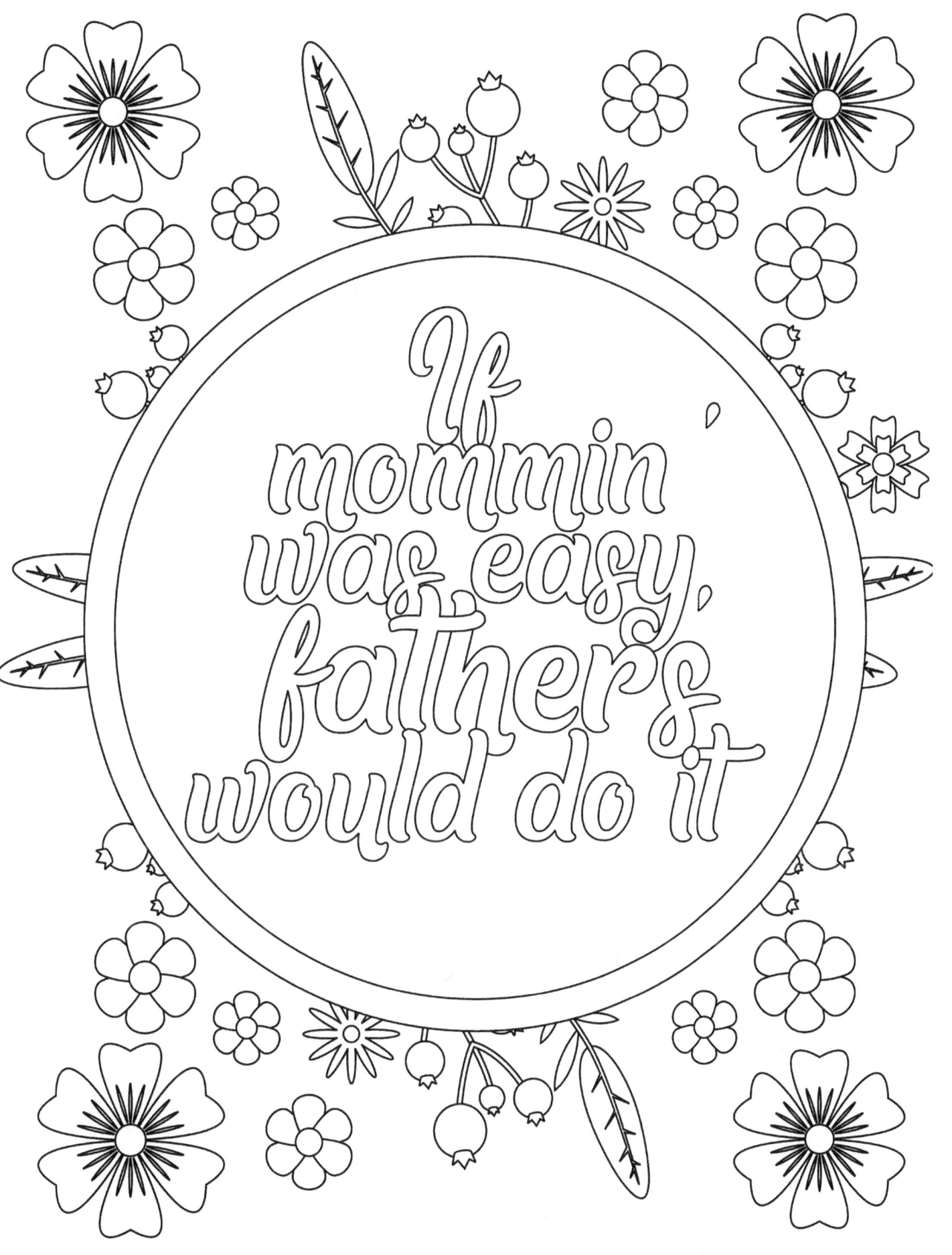

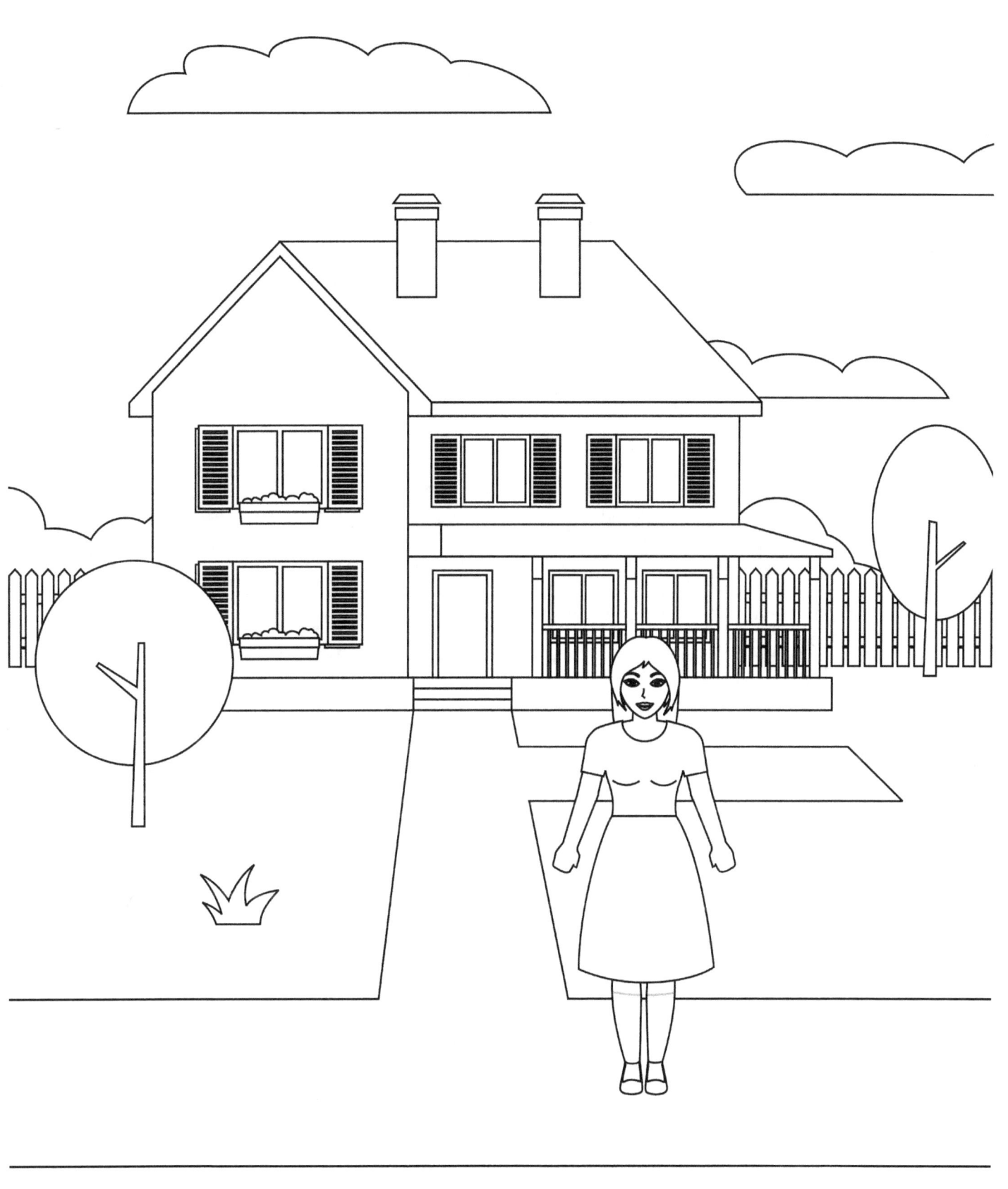

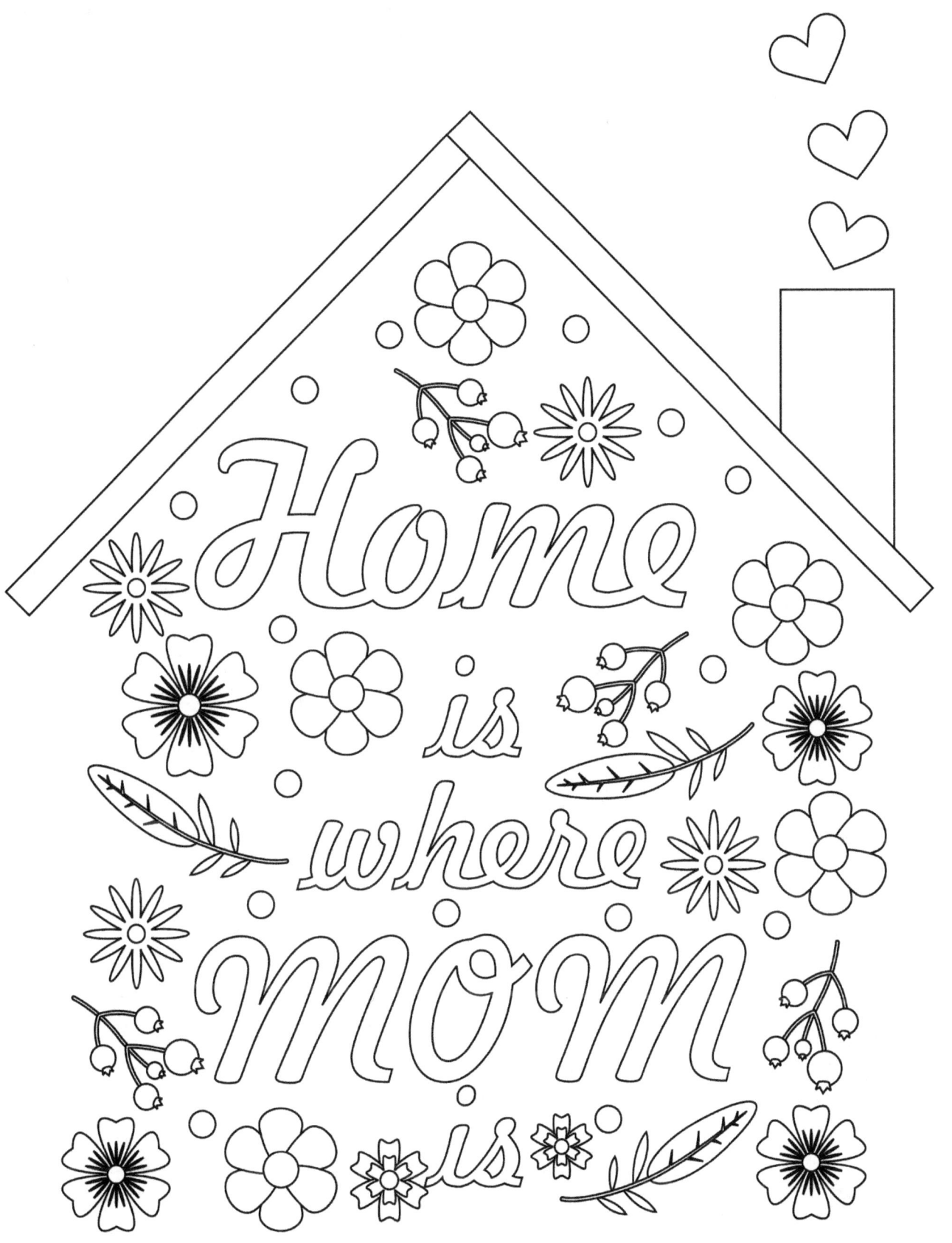

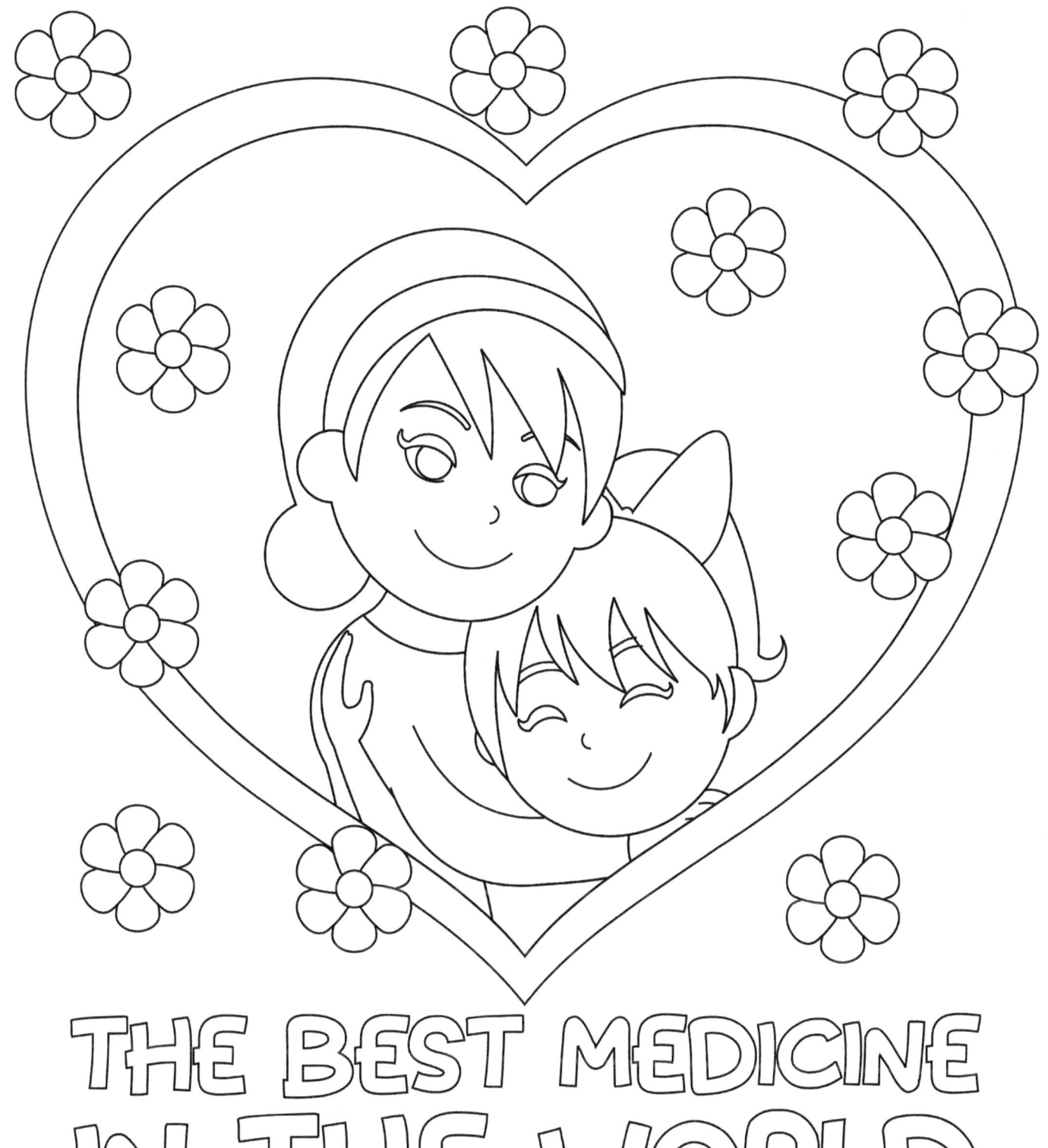

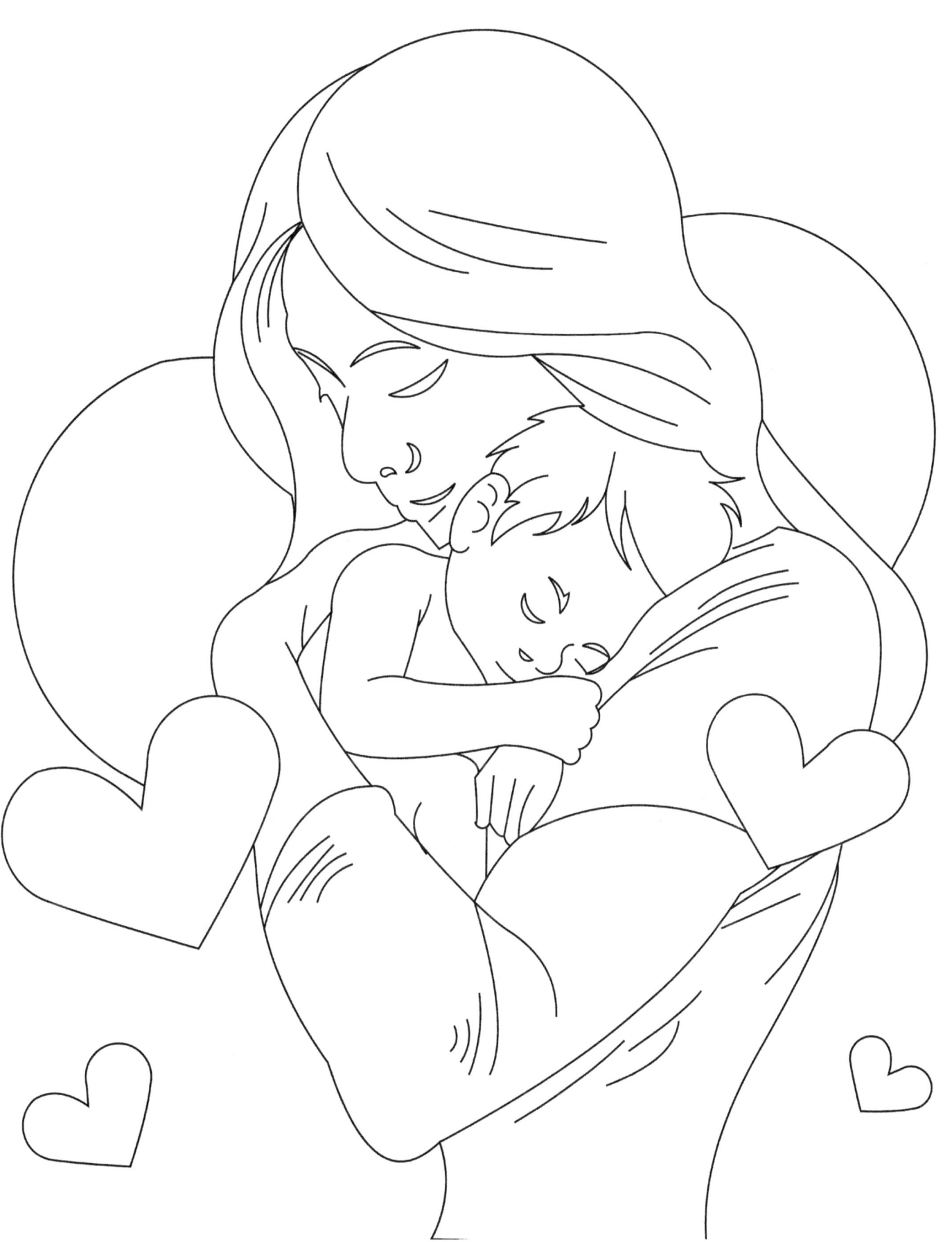

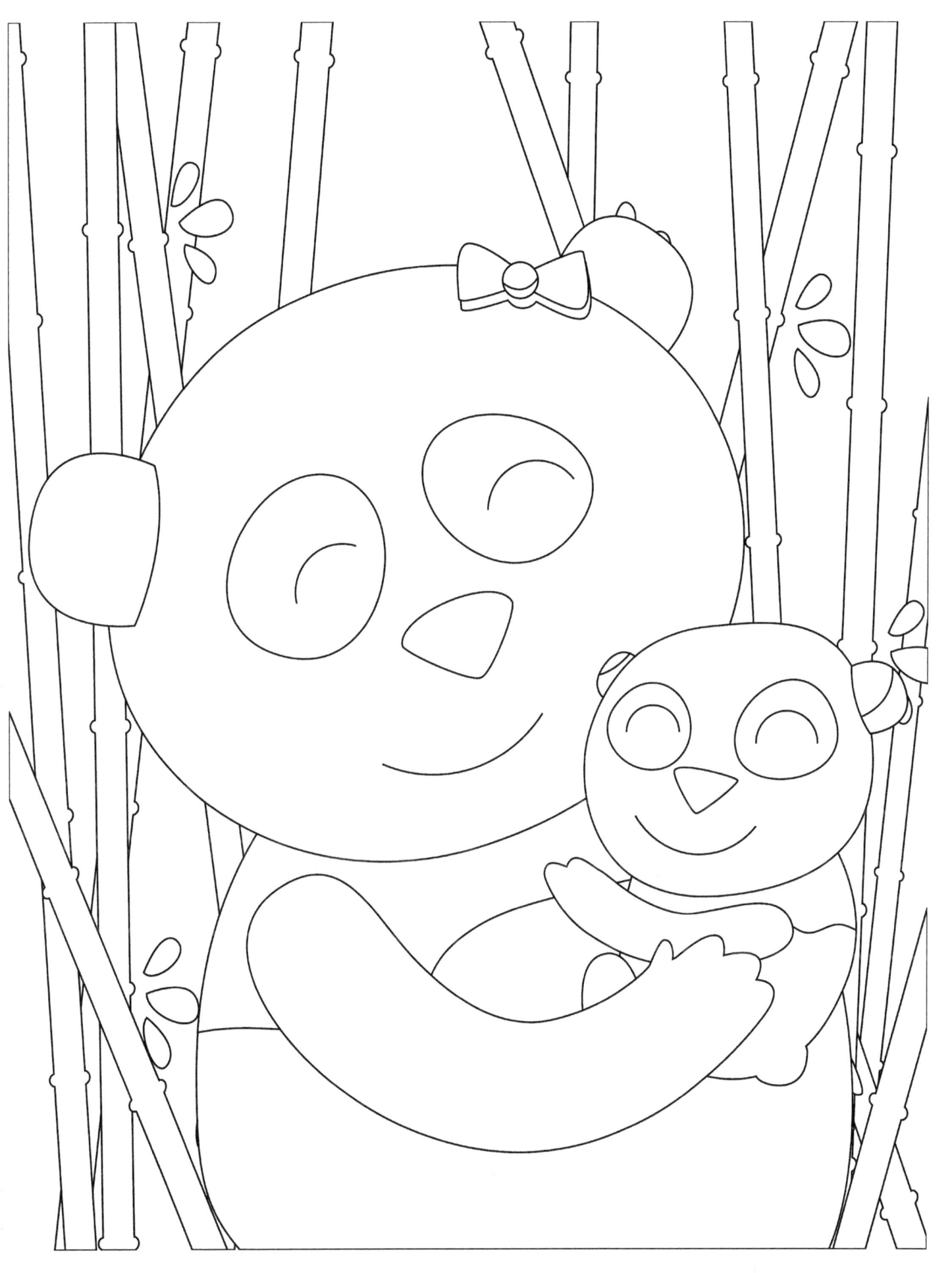

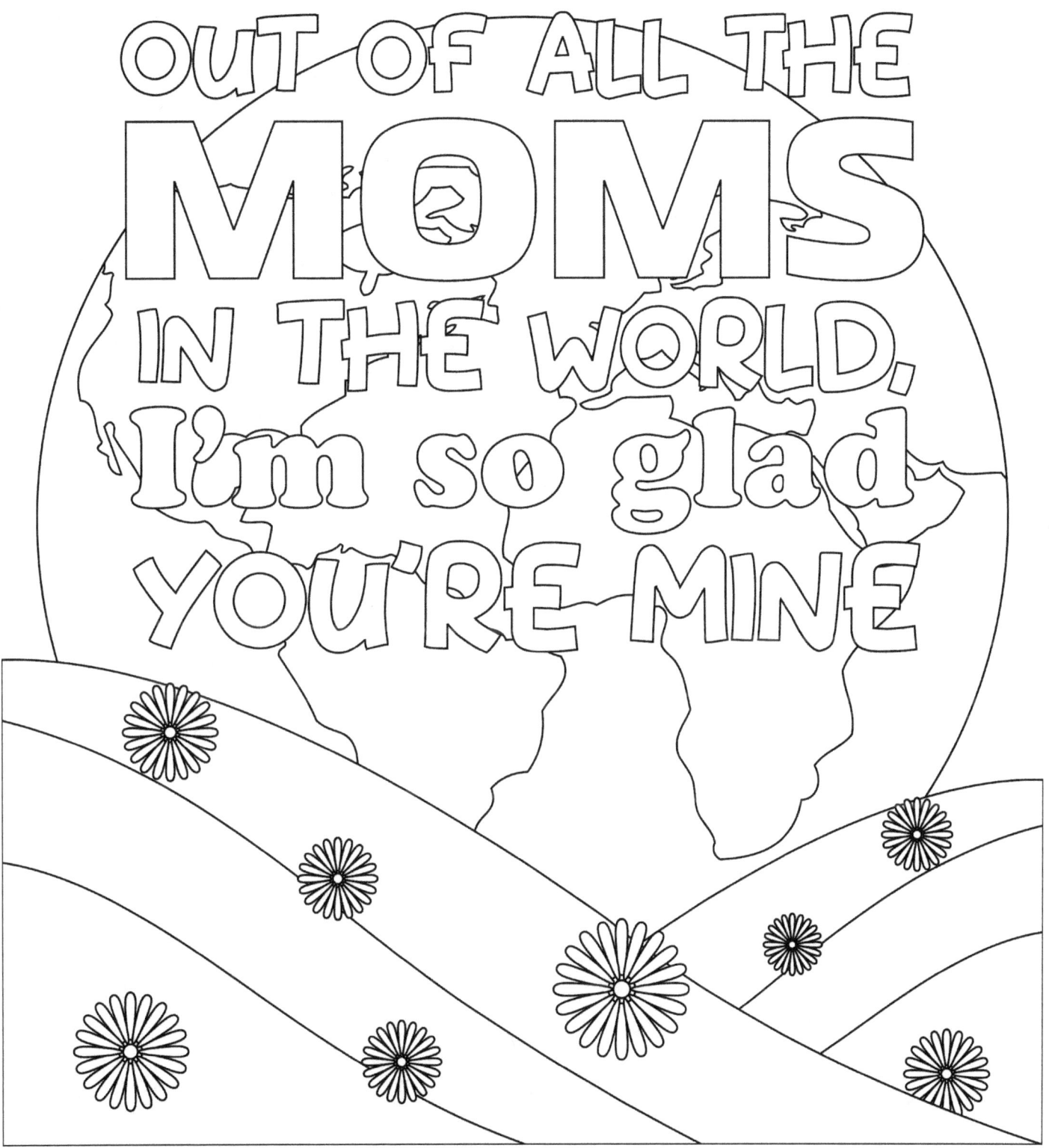

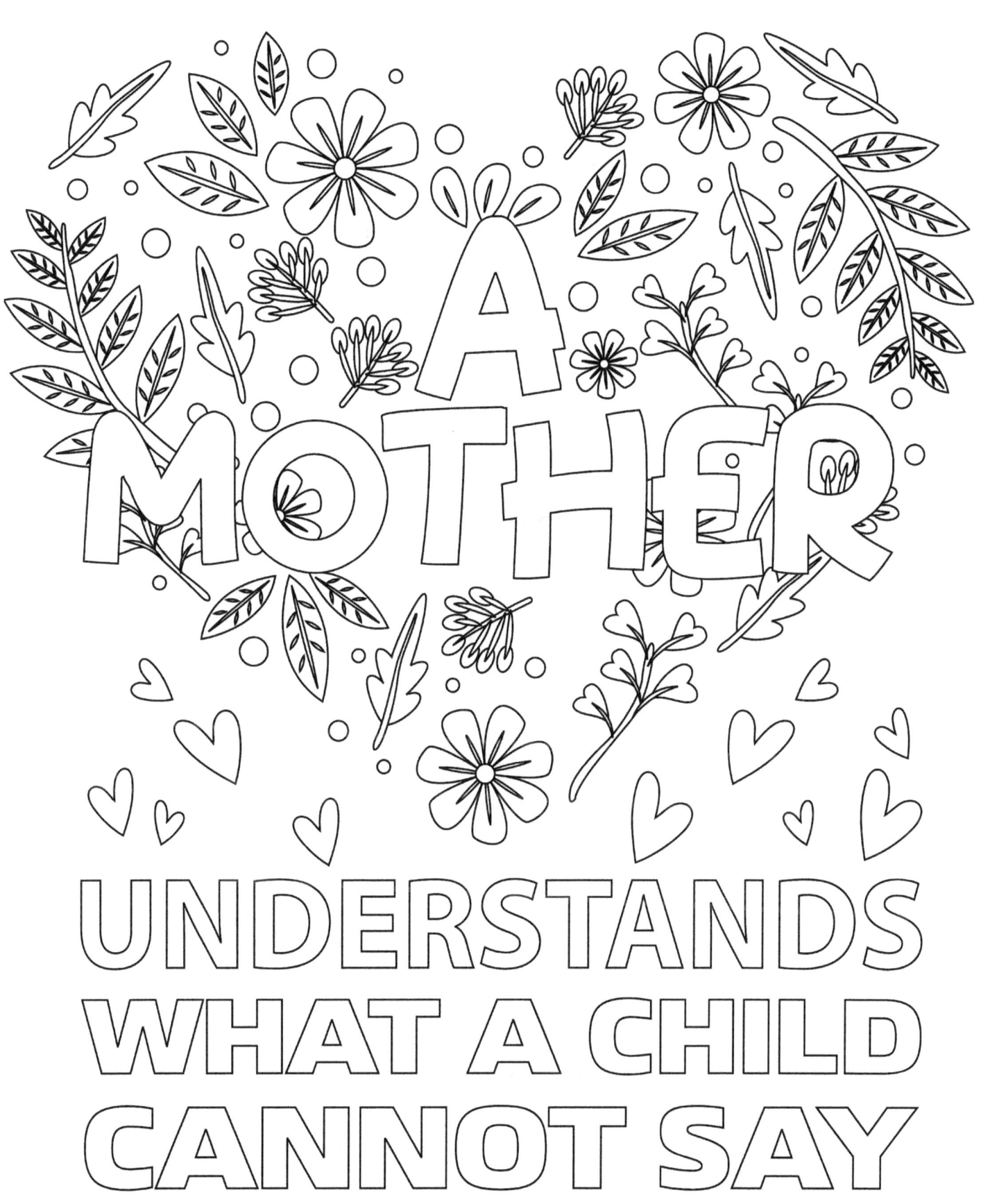

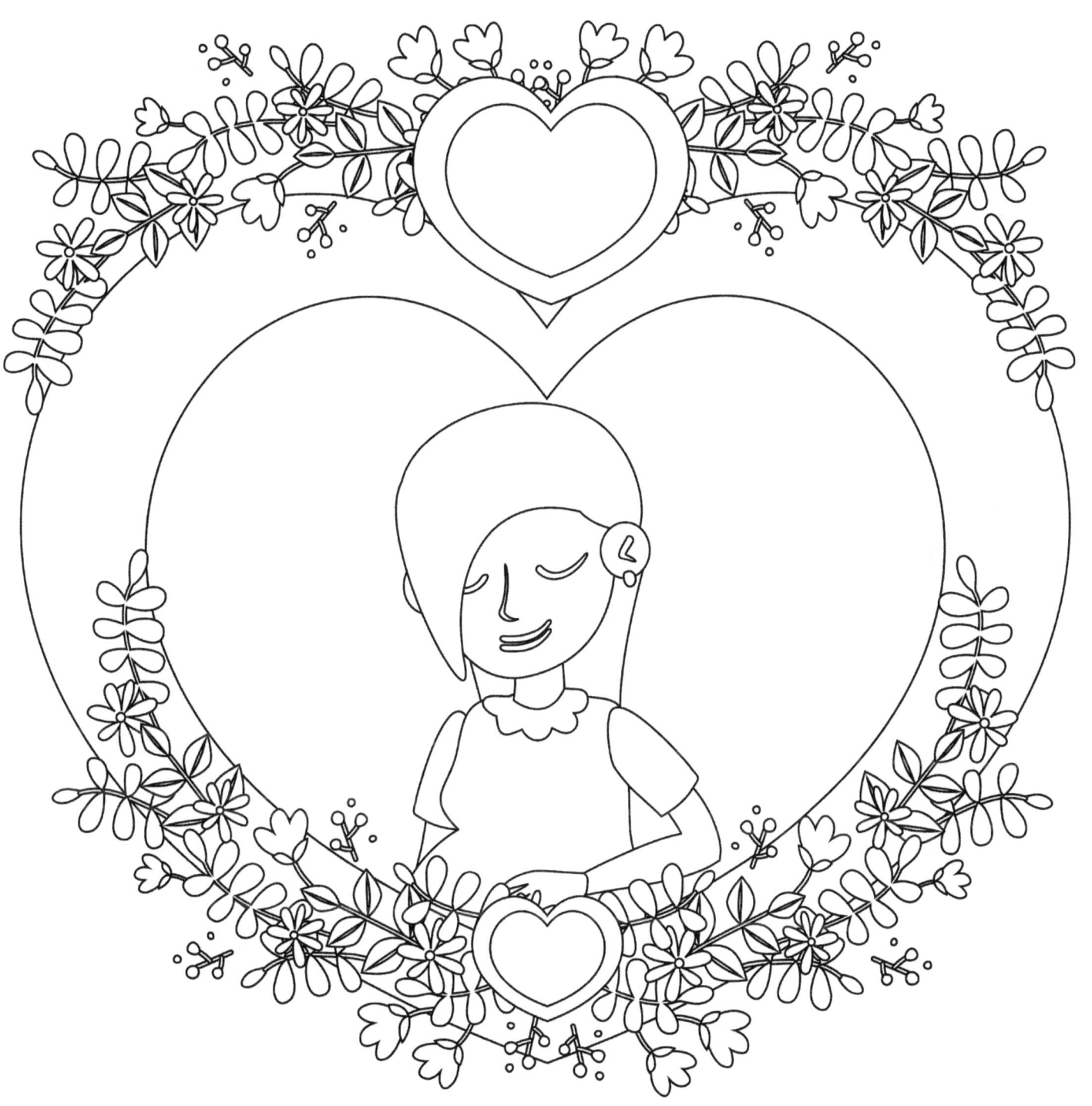

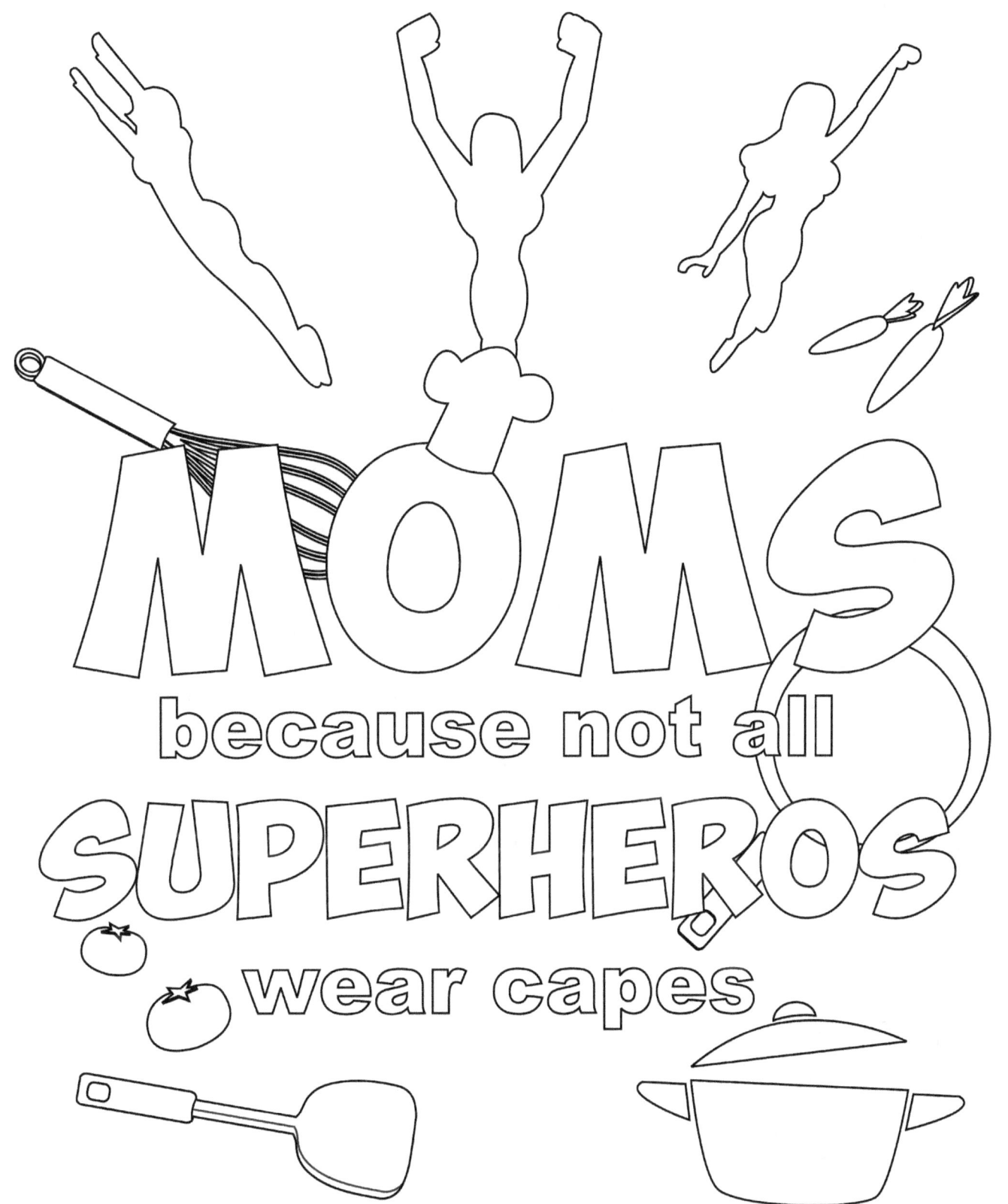

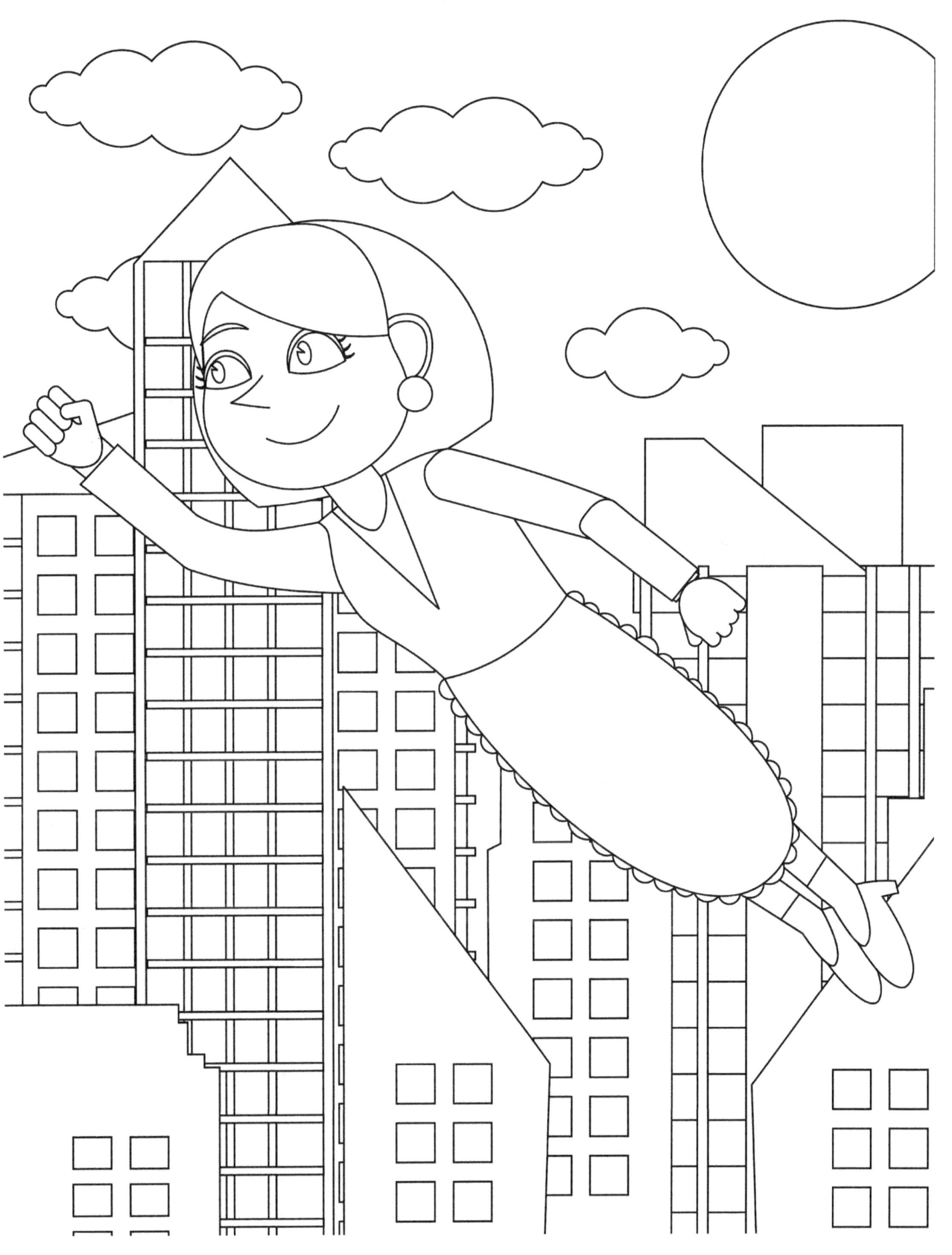

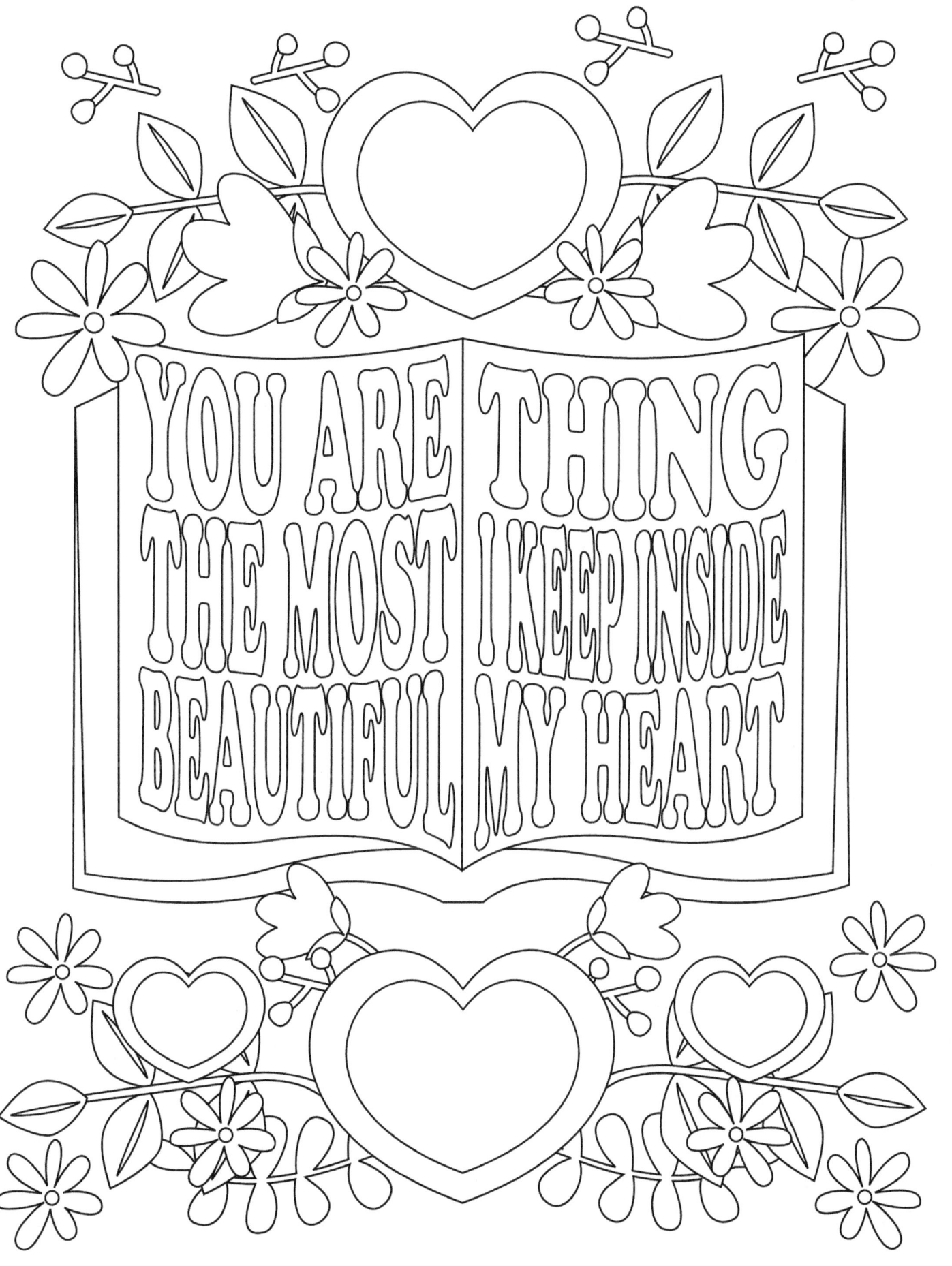

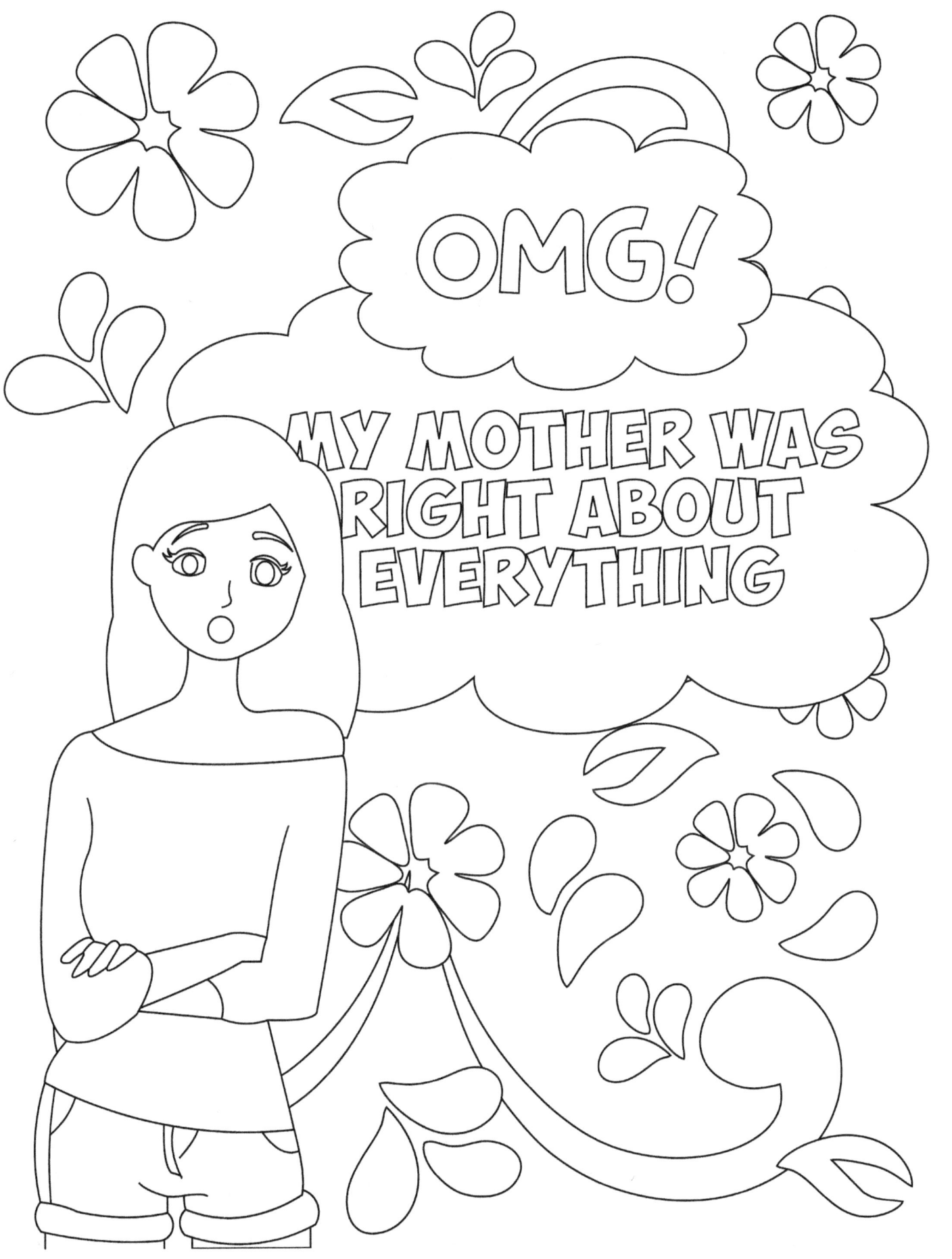

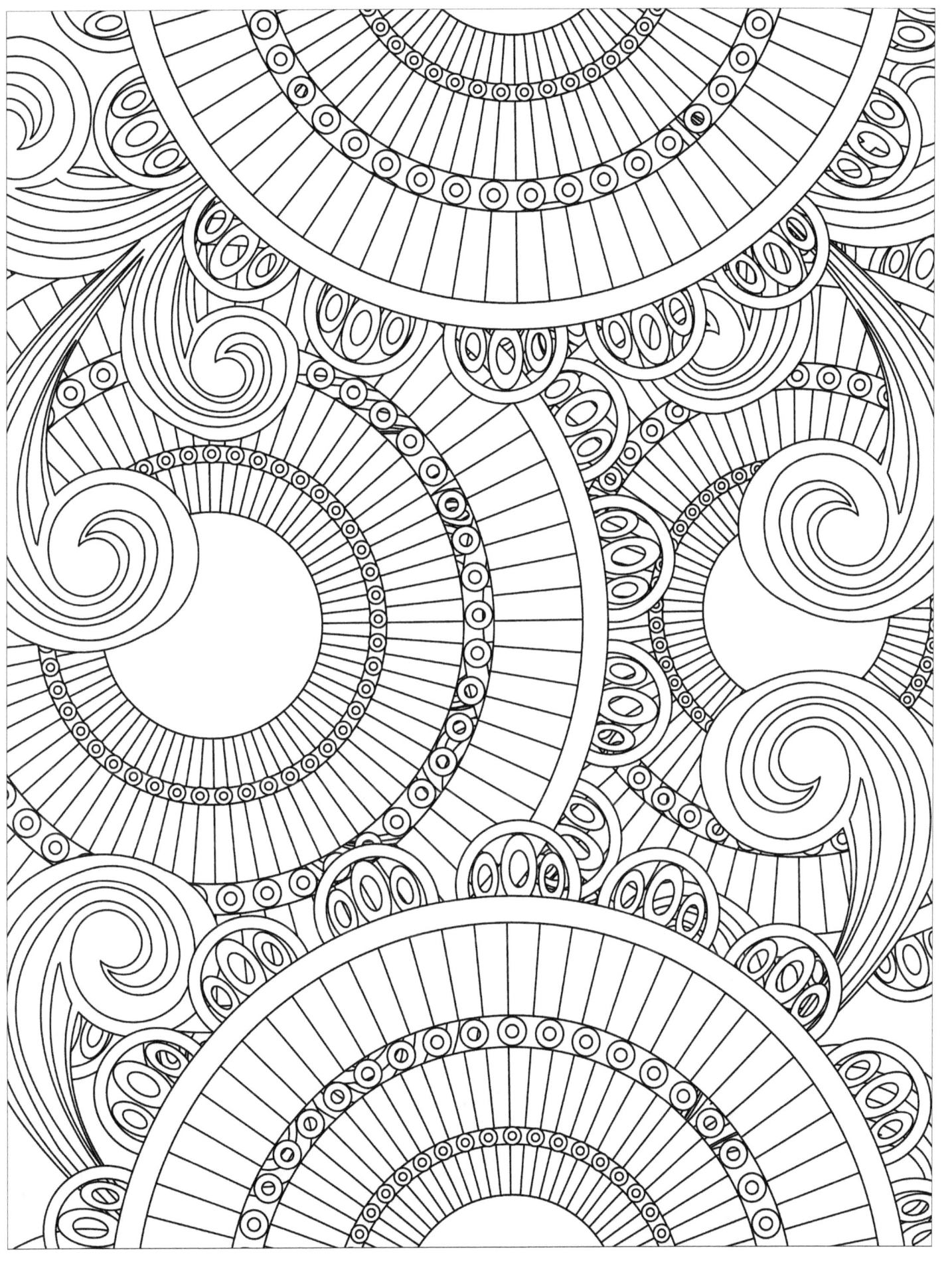

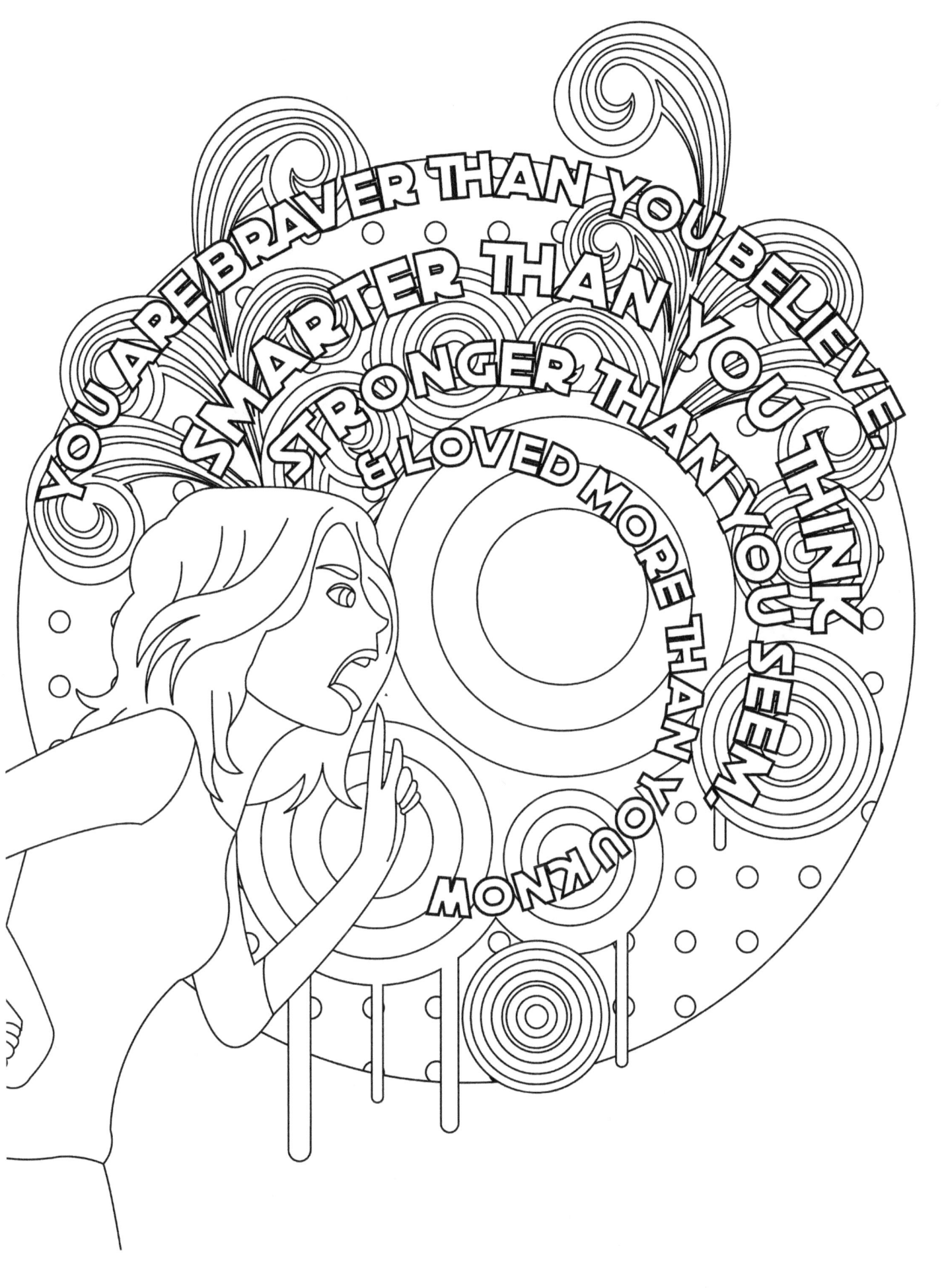

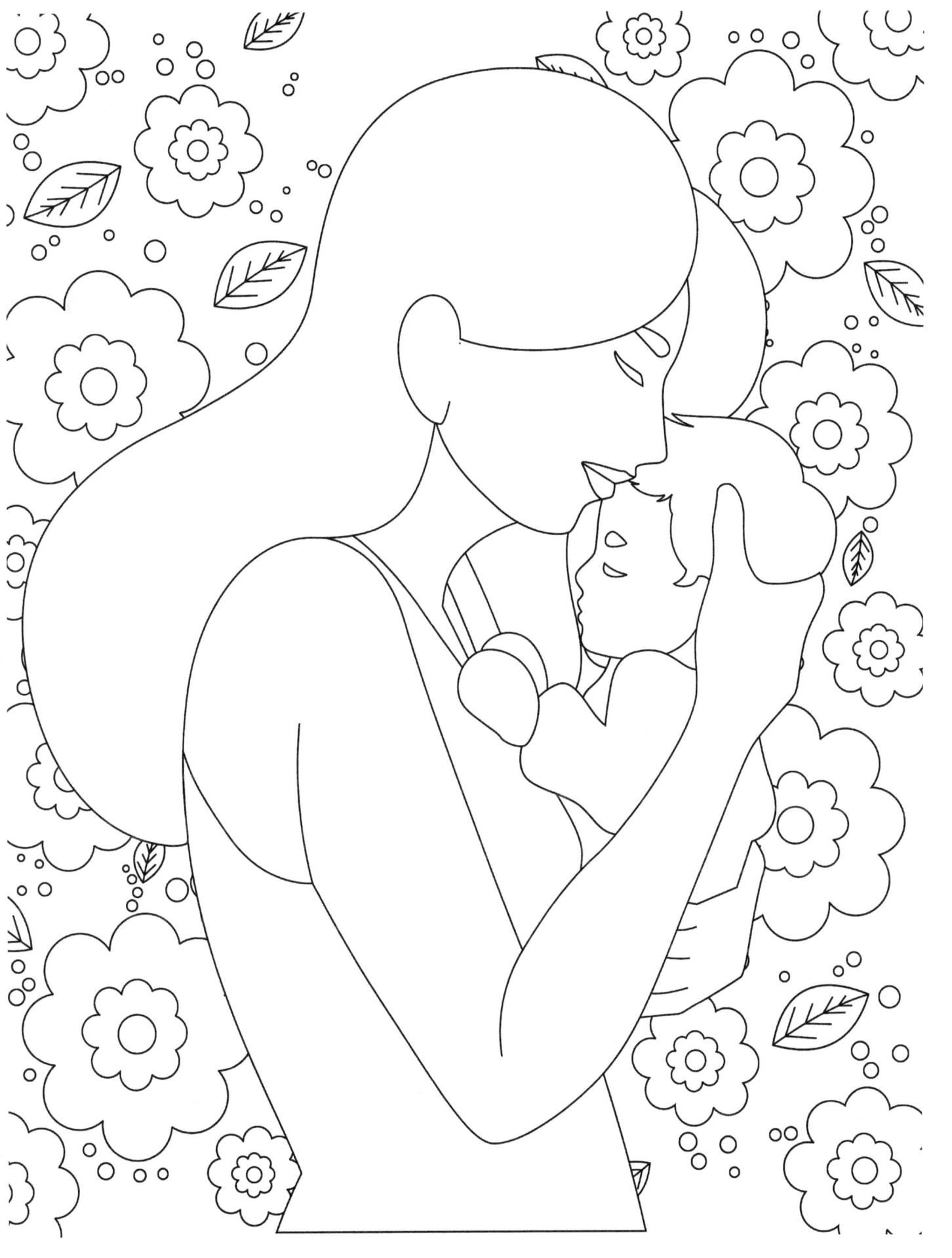

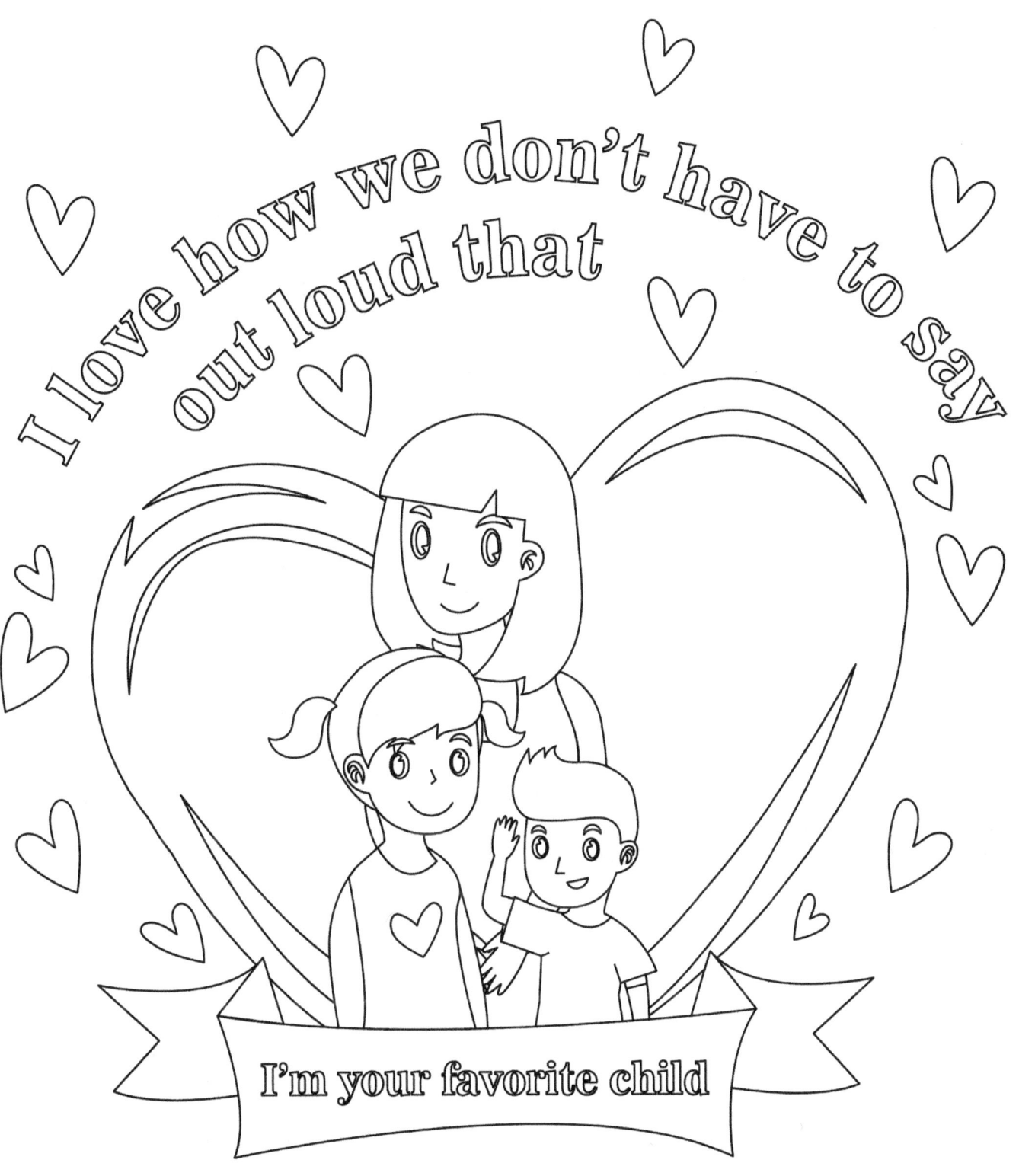

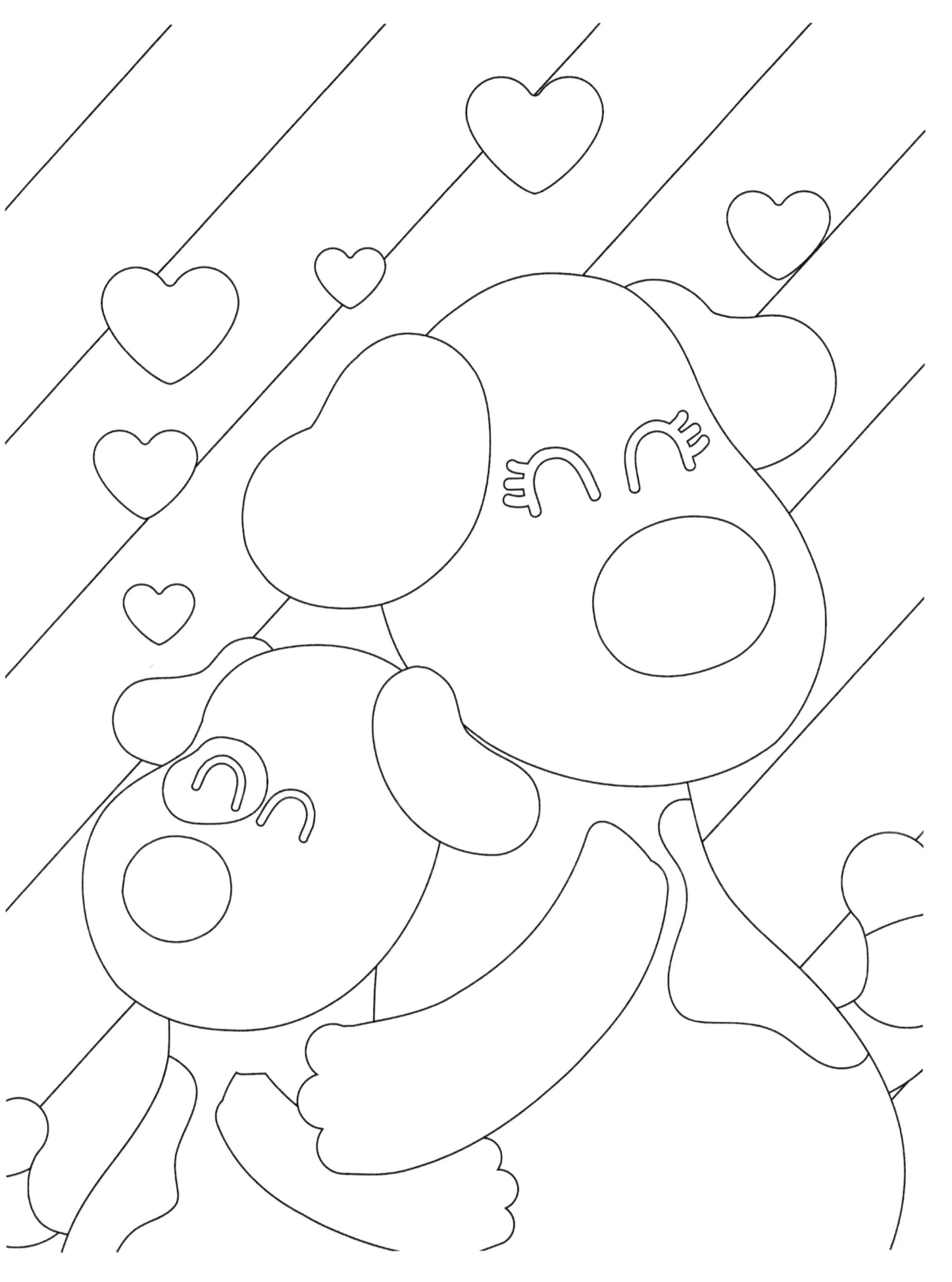

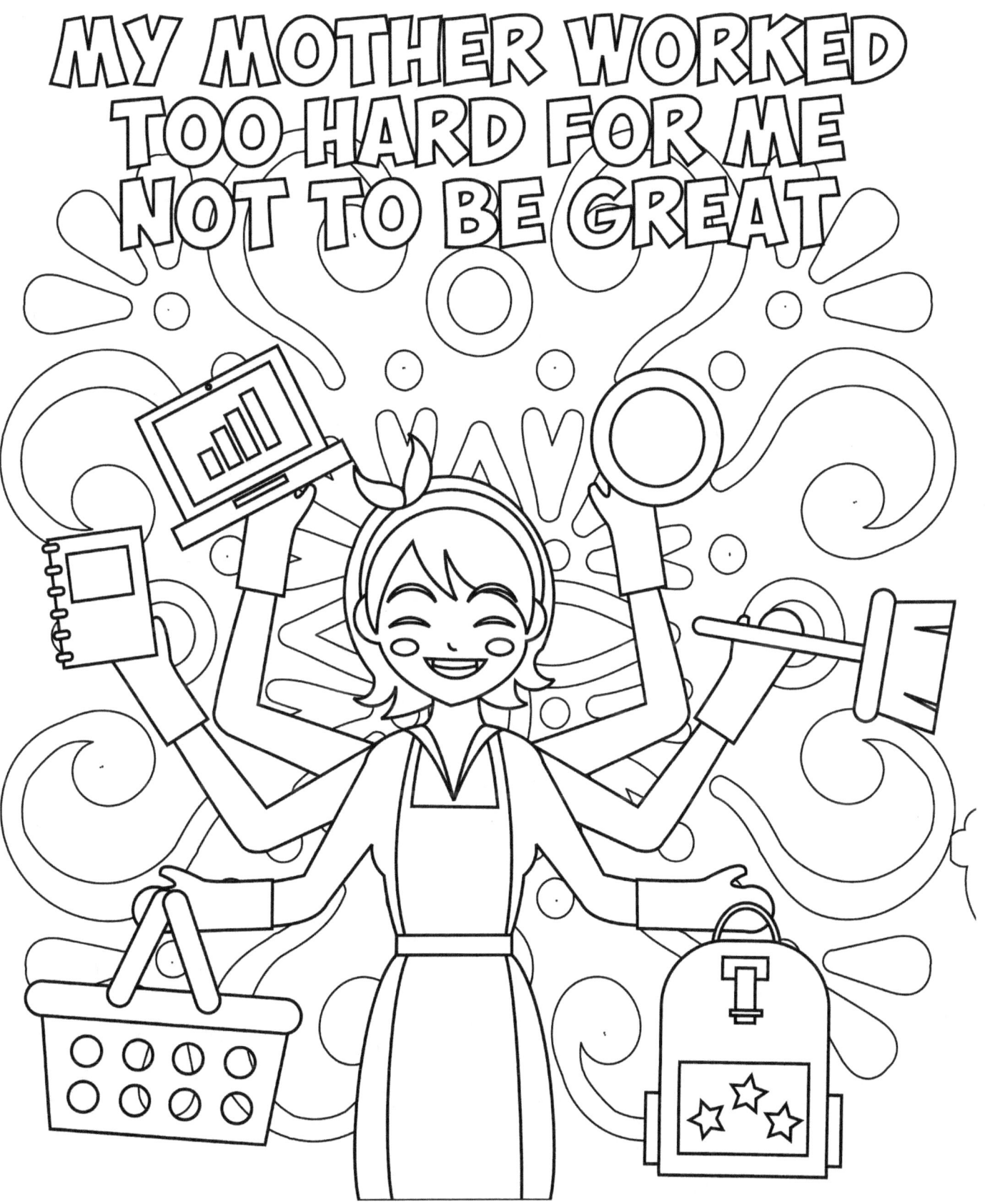

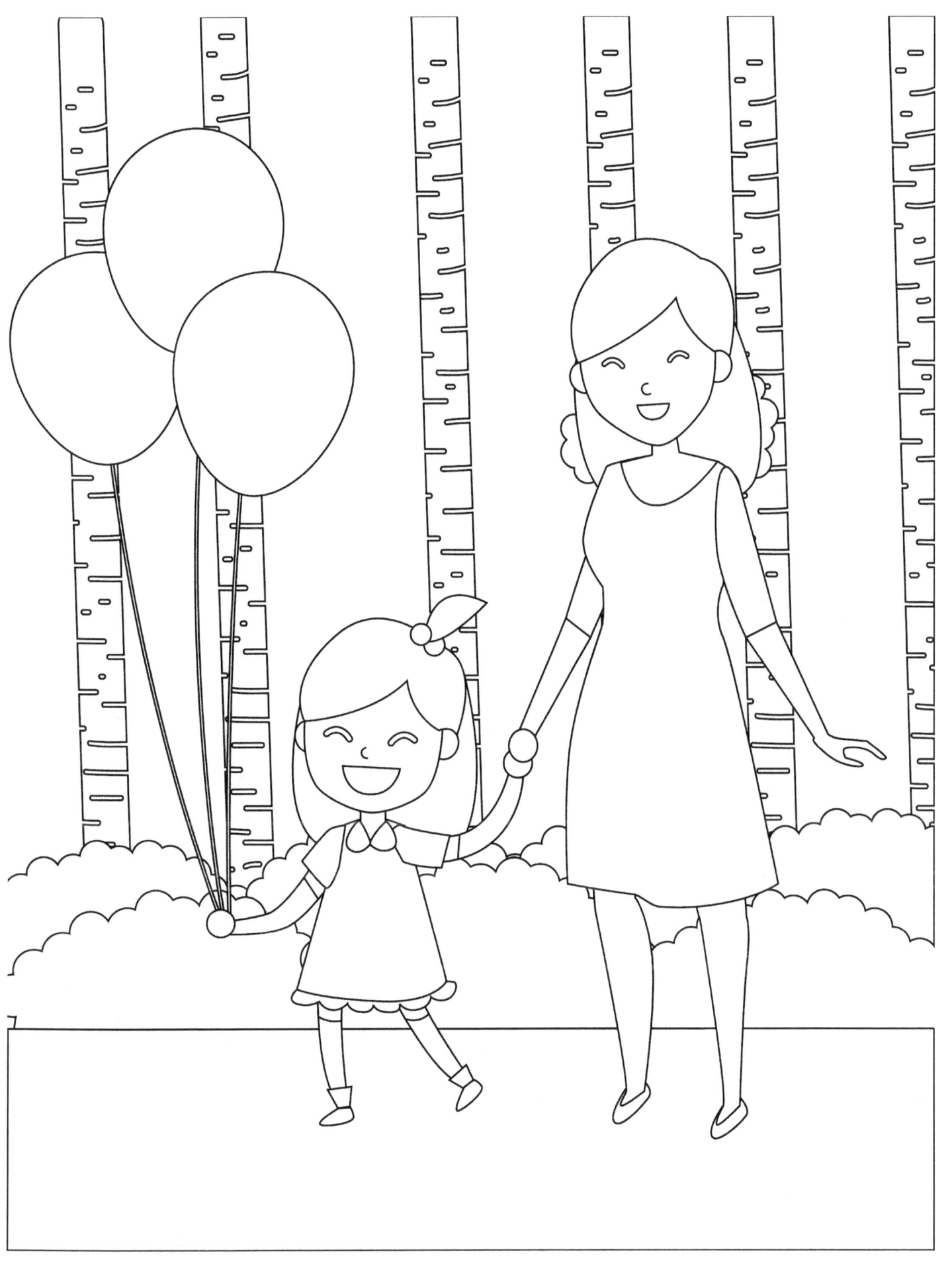